I Hear a Song in My Head

I Hear a Song in My Head

A Memoir in Stories of Love, Fear, Doctoring, and Flight

Nergesh Tejani, M.D.

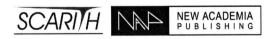

SCARITH · NEW ACADEMIA PUBLISHING

Washington, DC

Printed in the United States of America

Library of Congress Control Number: 2012934318

ISBN 978-0-9845832-7-0 paperback (alk. paper)

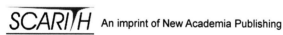 An imprint of New Academia Publishing

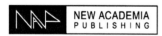 New Academia Publishing
PO Box 27420, Washington, DC 20038-7420
info@newacademia.com - www.newacademia.com

To all my beloveds

Contents

Reproduced with permission:

Tejani, Nergesh. Gentle Hands Lancet 1997; 349 (Issue 9064): 1562.

Tejani, Nergesh. Unspeakable Deeds Obstet Gynecol 2008; 111:187-188.

Tejani, Nergesh. Fistula Obstet Gynecol 2000; 96 1009-1010.

Acknowledgements

After my husband, Amir, died, the only times that I spent in relative peace were when I was asleep or writing of him. I chose to write about the most event-filled and exciting time of my life—the eleven years we spent in Kampala, Uganda, East Africa. This might be the only positive thing that was born as a result of his death—a celebration of those African years.

My thanks to Emily Pechefsky, that rigorous English scholar with whom I share two grandchildren. She read my writings with an unflinching eye and honest, sometimes ruthless, critiques. And in her acerbic manner, she convinced me that I had a voice that others may care to hear. And to Carol Sicherman who painstakingly edited my meandering thoughts. My thanks to Karen Getchell who carefully picked up after me.

And I thank Gareth Barberton, my co-trainee in Kampala and my companion in the London months. He asked, cajoled, commanded me to write of my life. And to do it fast or he may not be around to read the story.

Prologue

The White Coat

The date was December 19th, 1969. Late one velvet African night we returned home after an evening with friends at the Leopard's Lair—a Western-style nightclub with local spirit. The friends we had been with called later that night, telling us that Prime Minister Obote had been shot and injured. He was attending a political rally close to our home and someone, suspected to be a dispossessed Muganda, had tried to assassinate him. The bullet had gone through his jaw, and he had been taken to Mulago Hospital.

Next morning, I got a call from the small hospital where I worked. Mrs. Patel was in labor. She had regular contractions, reassuring fetal heart tones and was five centimeters dilated. I'm coming...I'm coming.

Got my six-year-old Rushna ready for school, took my three-year-old Cena across the road to nursery school and fed my one-year-old Sharyn. Combining work with being a mother was now natural and smooth.

I donned my white doctor's coat and took off in my sportsy Triumph, forgetting the events of the night before. The road to the hospital went past Mulago Hospital. I was stopped at a road block near the hospital by a clattering army presence. 'Out of your cars and open the trunk,' was the bark. Out of the car was fine, but I knew the trunk of my car did not open. A smallish knot formed in my upper abdomen.

An Indian couple climbed out of the van in front of me —a man and his diminutive wife, I assumed. Approaching them, bayonet poised, was an oversized human in polished boots and starched khakis.

'We were searched before,' whispered the woman in Swahili.

The man in the boots turned on her. She was no higher than his armpit. The handle of his bayonet cracked across her head and she lay quietly across the road. Her husband raised both his arms in a sign of surrender. A frozen scene before me—a raised lethal weapon, a tiny woman on the ground and her protector, pale and speechless.

I turned away. There was no question of helping. Also, 'boots' was walking toward me. I had a sickening remembrance of the unopenable trunk.

He took in my white coat.

'Good morning, doctor,' he said in Sandhurst inflections. 'I won't hold you up. Have a nice day.'

With a mechanical smile on my face, I fumbled into the car. I glanced at the savaged couple. The man was carrying his wife into the van.

Again I turned away. My powerful white coat could not help this hurt.

I arrived at my hospital. Was I the same person as before? To witness violence has to cause some shift in humors. To witness violence and not react—that must increase choler. To witness violence, rely on the protection of the white coat, the healer's symbol, and not react—a cult of barbarism.

I walked into Mrs. Patel's room. She was fully dilated and pushing. Relentless labor cares nothing for politics. Cares nothing for the wounded prime minister at Mulago Hospital shot by those he had excluded from power. Cares nothing for a slight woman felled in savagery.

I changed into scrubs, smiled. I let others exhort her to push... push. I could wait.

I waited for the scene of horror to pass. I am still waiting. Was the husband forever diminished in her eyes? Did she notice the woman in the white coat who made no move to help her? Did she go home and continue—prepare a meal, tend to her children, go to work? Did she start to fear a recalcitrant houseboy? Did her mind make preparations to leave the country, probably of her birth?

I see a little peep of scalp. Push, oh, push, that timeless chant. *Jor karo...sindika...empuja.* Words for the universally useful 'push' in many languages.

More dark hair asserted itself even between contractions. Mrs. Patel and family needed to know the exact time when the widest diameter of the head was delivered. The child's horoscope would be based on star relationships at that time. It is not the birth of the heart or gut but the brain that is crucial to this little one's future. A responsibility not taught in obstetric textbooks, noting the time of crowning of the head. Well, here it was. A dark wet head crowned by a halo of stretched maternal tissue. Crowned by its mother.

The baby girl slithered out. Pink and reactive. The family outside were silent when informed. Too well bred to be openly sad for yet another girl.

One said consolingly, *'Laxmi'*—'Wealth'.

There were tears in the new mother's eyes but she gathered her wiped baby to her breast and closed her eyes.

I changed back to street clothes, donned my white coat and re-entered a changed world.

As things wind down for me, I look back on all the stories I was privileged to be part of. Some of the passport one gets when there is an M.D. tacked onto your name whether in New York or Uganda. Stories worth telling.

My story starts at the end of my Obstetrics and Gynecology registrarship in Bombay, India, where I lived, went to medical school and married and covers the eleven years we lived in Uganda, East Africa, and our first year in the U.S. I included this last year because at the end of it, Idi Amin, who 'reigned' in Uganda after a military coup, had a dream in which he was commanded to banish the Asian population of Uganda. This dream and order was announced on August 9th, 1972, with a deadline for leaving three months later on November 9th. In October and the first week of November 1972, our extended family arrived in bits and pieces on the shores of North America, to be welcomed by us who had arrived here by chance, whim and luck the year before.

ONE

Amir

To understand my life I have to tell you about him. In brief, in short, in staccato. Our beginnings could not have been more different. His father was an impoverished teacher at the Aga Khan School in tiny one-street Sultanhamood in Kenya.

Decades later Amir and I visited this outpost and tears clouded his eyes. His memory of a grand and spacious living had been magnified and beautified by time. They lived in a small section of the mosque area, and the schoolhouse was in an adjoining room. This time around he stared with disbelief at the small living area

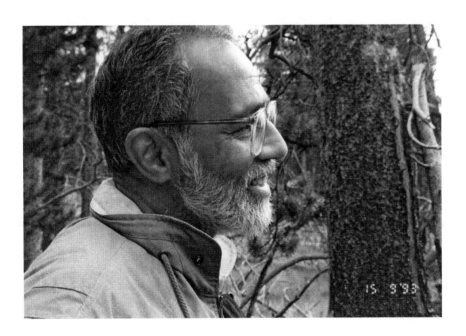

and the corrugated tin roof that thundered in the rain. A gracious Swahili lady took us around and said she remembered Amir's father. When we looked at her disbelievingly, she proved it by telling us of something that she could only have known from that time. His father officiated as the elder in the mosque, and all cash collections were hidden under a loose stone flag in the room that served as school and mosque. Both Amir and she laughed at the memory and together pried open the stone to reveal the secret place beneath. Quite empty and no cash there today.

Many were the stories of their poverty. No shoes till the age of seven or eight. And even then they were bought several sizes too large so as to serve long years of growth. Shorts only—no long trousers. Butter once a week, which had to be fetched from the next village miles away. An expedition taken on by foot or bicycle. Breaking an article of crockery would be met with fierce reprisals from his mother because of the difficulty of replacing it.

And yet his family life was dear and utterly happy. A world away I was being reared by my loveless grandmother after my mother died in that 'maximum city,' Bombay. Middle-class and westernized, but cold and remote. Passion was unseemly and never displayed, except in the form of a constantly angry grandmother. She had no stomach for child-rearing and let me and my two sisters know.

And then there was his religious life. He was born an Ismaili, a Shiite sect, followers of a living Imam, the Aga Khan. As a young boy the Ismaili-ness of his life entered into daily doings. The mosque was a place of worship, a social spot. And life revolved around it. We often laughed at the seriousness with which he had taken his youthful mosque duties—later he was to become as derelict as I. His first disenchantment came when he applied for a scholarship to go to college and medical school in Bombay and was refused it in spite of his academic achievements. The scholarship was awarded to a relative of the presiding official. When Amir went to make his case, he was told to tag along and be a doormat to the official and maybe his case would be reopened. He refused and obtained a more general Uganda government scholarship. That was the beginning of his religious unraveling. In another part of the world, the superficialities and rituals of the Parsi Zoroastrian religion surrounded me and I, from a very young age, refused its protection.

The family moved to Singida, a tiny township in Tanganyika. Amir's father gave up teaching to start a business so as to provide for his fast-growing family. He opened a general store in Singida that sold everything from socks to grain and yards and yards of 'maricani' (from America), a khaki poplin fabric that was stitched into pants by a resident tailor working a Singer foot-peddled sewing machine on the verandah.

Time came when Amir had to leave home to go to high school, the Aga Khan School in Dar-es-Salaam. As he later watched his grandchildren not need to tie shoelaces because of the velcro revolution, he remembered how he left for school with his first pair of shoes, unable to tie his laces. He excelled in spite of the oft-applied rod, inedible food and many cruelties. Once when they were being taught about the Taj Mahal—Indian history and geography in Africa—his most favorite and beloved teacher told of its romance and read odes to it and to love in general. This teacher was soon removed because of his romantic real life. The replacement who met the approval of the higher-ups, when describing the Taj Mahal, made the children memorize its dimensions, the number of archways and other cold realisms.

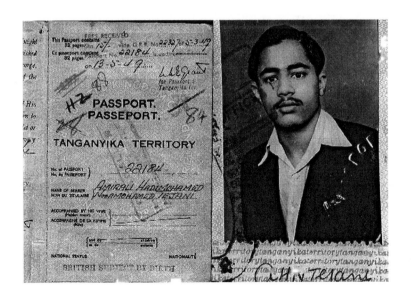

A major event in the erstwhile boys school was the admission of girls. It seemed to me that the initial group of 'trail-blazer' girls were largely ornamental and were constantly being asked to sing popular Indian songs for the boys. None passed the qualifying exams. One caught Amir's eye and her golden voice filled his ears. One song, a sentimental but haunting one, telling of how she would live and die unseen in his street, he remembered, and often sang under his breath. Where did his thoughts fly when he remembered that old song?

He made his first Indian Ocean crossing in 1949 at the age of sixteen. This was to be the first of many such journeys from the east coast of Africa to Bombay. He traveled in the cheapest part of the liners that ploughed these seas several levels below the deck. While all around him were in miseries with *mal-de-mer*, he stocked up on his ever-favorite Kit-Kat chocolates and made them last the seven days crossing. He said he had to consume them 'to prevent them from melting' in the furnace heat of the underbelly of the ship. At different times during these crossings, the ships stopped at Seychelles, Madagascar or Mauritius, all of which he roamed. One of the Seychelles Islands is Amirante, no doubt named for him. Lorenço Marques, now Maputo in Mozambique, was another name that he evoked in romantic memory of those ocean journeys.

In Bombay he started studies at the then-elite Elphinstone College. A few miles away I was attending the much inferior Jai Hind College. I had not found my star yet, and organic chemistry left me in disarray. Two years later we both were admitted to the Grant Medical College, he on merit and I on questionable merit but helped by the alumnus status of my father.

I found my muse in medicine. And in a way he did, too. I roared through at the top of my class. And he thoroughly enjoyed those young years which were there to enjoy. He had a group of male friends with whom he played poker till the wee hours of the morning while drinking bootleg liquor in prohibition Bombay. A succession of nurses enjoyed his fun and company. In the third year of five-year medical school, he excelled in one examination—Pharmacology—and that is when I first noticed him.

Another highlight of his distinctly non-academic medical school years was the famous 'SJ Mehta trial.'

SJ Mehta was an irascible surgeon in the old school mold. He terrorized and even brutalized medical students, specially those in the 'Amir mold.' He would walk into surgery—gallbladder was his special favorite—with a lighted cigarette between his lips. If ash fell into the open belly, he claimed it was sterile and stimulated healing. A 'ward boy' stood behind him at the operating table with the only function of removing and replacing the cigarette from his mouth. From his mouth would also emanate the vilest curses directed toward his forever-inept house officers. They did nothing that satisfied his sense of perfection, and knuckle bashing with a variety of surgical instruments was background music to all his surgery.

Amir and his pals organized a mock trial accusing SJ of crimes including physical and emotional assault, and defamation directed against medical students. Amir appointed himself the chief prosecutor with a team of assistants. SJ gamely consented to appear but refused the offer of one of the nerdy male students to be his defense counsel. He would, of course, conduct his own defense.

Several traumatized medical students were rehearsed and brought in as witnesses against SJ. One stated that a naso-gastric tube had been forced into his stomach as punishment for not knowing the pH of gastric juice. SJ's defense was that this student would never ever forget the indications for the use of a naso-gastric tube and thus he had done the student a favor in teaching him an unforgettable lesson.

Predictably, I did not attend Amir's glorious moment in this event, which I thought too frivolous a waste of my time. But all accounts of it for days after reported a coup decisively won for the students by Amir Tejani.

Our five years ended in grueling exams in seven clinical disciplines. Each had written (essay type, not multiple choice) and oral examinations involving actual patients. The whole process was spread over a month, and after that experience all future exams paled into insignificance. The pharmacology star did not repeat his brilliance, but I did excel. Was it that that attracted him? He claims it was not my brain but only my legs that drew him in toward me. But it occurred soon after the examination results that we became an item, a team. All our acquaintances predicted a short affair because of our outward incompatibilities and dissimilarities. Well, it lasted forever. Literally till death did us part.

He decided on pediatrics as his specialty and entered an internship on one of the busy pediatric units at our campus. There were so few real teachers at the time. But the junior attending on his unit was a slim quiet man, devoted to children with an encyclopedic knowledge--Dr. Wagle, forever remembered by Amir.

While working on this, his first pediatrics job, he started a habit which I thought awful but would always earn him people who adored him beyond everything and those who could not stand him. He played flagrant favorites. A little girl, Nimmi, stole his heart away. She was a long-term resident in the hospital with tubercular meningitis and liquid eyes and a smile to die for. We never went anywhere without him bringing back a gift for Nimmi—often a jasmine bracelet. No matter how late we would be back from our evening roamings, he would pop into the pediatrics ward to give it to her. Jasmine does not last beyond a few hours but Nimmi was his forever.

We interned for six months in one of the major specialties and then three months in a minor one. He did a minor in Dermatology or 'skin,' as it was disparagingly called. The chief on 'skin' was a romantic eccentric, Dr. L., who made instant diagnoses and never stopped to explain the reasoning behind his decision. The applications and management for all the diseases he diagnosed were the same, so it really did not make that much difference. Dr. L. always had a certain rose-like aura about him. On asking about the rose smell, I was told that every day on his way to work he stopped his chauffeur-driven Mercedes Benz at one of the row of ear-cleaning establishments in Bhindi Bazaar just outside the main hospital gate.

In response to a honk of the horn, the impoverished *kansaf* (*kan*=ear *saf*=clean) rushed out to Dr. L., still seated in the double or triple parked car, with home-made Q-tips and hot oil. He poured the oil into Dr. L's wax-filled ears, rolled his (the doctor's) head around a bit and then scraped out the oil and wax with the Q-tip. Following this, a rose-attar drenched clean Q-tip was placed under the outer fold of each ear. Dr. L. often arrived at the clinic with these Q-tips still sticking out of his ears, and a peon would help remove them before he started his morning of snap diagnoses. What chance did his interns have of learning any real dermatology?

It was now early 1958. Letters arrived from Amir's family in Africa. By this time they had moved to Kampala, Uganda. His father had started a business in this, the largest city in Uganda— not yet the capital. Once again, this time in the suitcase business, he did not prosper and thought this was the perfect time for Amir to return and start a practice in the space he had used as his store. It was time for Amir to come home after these long student years and take over the responsibility of helping support this large family. His father and mother had given him the best of opportunity to educate himself, and now it was time to start earning a living.

I never saw the letters between him and his parents, but I know there was no argument, and I and he accepted it as inevitable. I had just started a two-year senior training position in Obstetrics and Gynecology and did not doubt that I should complete it even though this advanced training would not be accepted toward the British boards that were required in Uganda. Perhaps we both thought we needed to contemplate things before making the plunge. I remember and know his reasoning more than mine. He had to go back, start his practice, move the family to a larger house—they lived in 'blue room,' a two-roomed apartment for the entire family of parents and nine children. During these two years apart, he did all this and the family moved into an independent house in 'Madras Gardens' in the Indian section of Kampala.

I remember my own resolve wavering in those two years but he never faltered and at the end of the two years was back in Bombay to start our time together as he had always planned.

TWO

The Early Kampala Years

1959—We get married

November 1959. At the end of my two-year registrarship—a senior training position in Obstetrics and Gynecology at Bai Motlabai Hospital in the JJ Hospital Group in Bombay—I was to sit for the Indian board examinations in Obstetrics and Gynecology. To my chagrin, my thesis was not accepted and I could not appear for the test. Looking back now, I see that it was an unacceptable thesis reflecting no understanding of what research entailed. There was also a singular lack of guidance to put me on track. I recall it was a treatise on ectopic gestation with no hypothesis, no stated purpose, no method section and therefore no results. It was just a description taken from common sources.

I was shaken. Everything else academic had just been too easy. I called Amir in Kampala, a call that had to go through the telephone operators in India and Uganda who conversed loudly and impatiently, one in Hindi and the other in Swahili. After several minutes of no comprehension, miraculously I heard his voice at the other end. His solution was typical. The board examiners knew nothing. The only solution was for him to fly over and for us to get married. It seemed like a splendid cure for everything.

There was a hitch—he was an Ismaili, a sub-sect of Moslem Shiites, and I was born a Parsi Zoroastrian, both selective and exclusive religions practiced by our families. These old religions are intertwined from antiquity.

The Parsis are members of the oldest, possibly 5,000-year-old, monotheistic religion following the prophet Zarathustra—

unrelated to Nietzsche—also called Zoroaster. Past glories climaxed in the Zoroastrian Emperor Darius, whose kingdom stretched over the Mediterranean, Red and Caspian Seas to the Indian Ocean. Alexander of Macedonia soon demolished this expanse and in 800 A.D., the Arabs overran the area. Many Zoroastrians, who were now concentrated in Persia, present-day Iran, converted to Islam. A small group assembled at the Straits of Hormuz at the junction of the Persian Gulf and the Indian Ocean and set sail in three sailing boats. Winds and chance brought them to the island of Diu, from whence they sailed to the Indian mainland and arrived at Sanjan on the west coast of India. The King of Sanjan sent them a cup filled to the brim with milk, indicating there was no room. In reply, they added a spoonful of sugar without spilling a drop. The king, impressed by their wit, allowed them to land, provided they only practiced their religious rites after dark so as not to influence the natives.

In India the Parsis (*Pars*, from Persia) lived quietly as farmers and small business people. Making country liquor was a common business, and one line of my forebears were called Daruvala (*daru*, alcohol). The Daruvala men were a jolly group who often came to Bombay to see the big city and respectfully visit my father, the only doctor in that clan. The Parsis lived quietly, causing no waves for almost a thousand years, till the British landed in India.

The British had a mixed reception amongst the diverse Indian population. However, with the Parsis there was no ambiguity. They welcomed the British with open arms and avidly identified with and absorbed their mores, language, literature and culture. It was as though they had been living under duress with the 'natives' and suddenly found their soul mates. They rapidly became negotiators between the British and the Indians. In return, the Parsis were regarded with trust almost, but not completely, equivalent to fellow Britishers, and indispensable when dealing with the incomprehensible natives.

The years of the British Raj were the halcyon days for the Parsis. With time and the new empowerment, they established themselves as master ship-builders, industrialists, educators, heads of business conglomerates and philanthropists. A whole city, Jamshedpur, was built around the Tata Steel Mills, named after Jamshedji Tata.

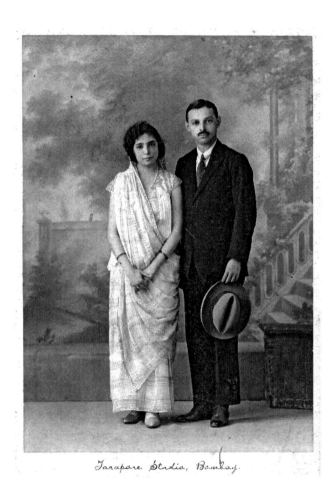

Tarapore Studio, Bombay.

Bombay's first hospital for the indigent—the JJ Hospital—was built supported by the philanthropy of Jamshedji Jeejiboy, also a Parsi. Its affiliation with the Grant Medical College resulted in the first medical school established in India. My father graduated from this school in 1919, and I and Amir in 1956.

I was born in 1933 in Bombay and for the first six years of my life moved to various military stations with my father Kaikhushru Manekji Bharucha, a doctor in the Royal Army Medical Corps, my mother Tehmina née Bode and my older sister Perrin. Old rambling colonial houses in Ambala, Lahore, Amritsar and Dalhousie were our homes, with Perrin changing schools frequently.

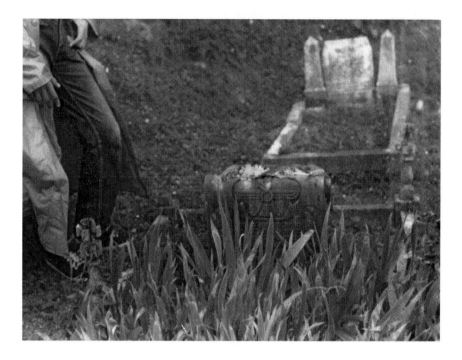

In 1939 when I was six, my younger sister Shirin, six months, and my older sister, twelve years, our mother Tehmina died of typhoid fever while we were on holiday in Mussoorie, in the foothills of the Himalayas. Her grave lies on a terraced misty hill with irises thrusting out of her breast through the broken slab, in the company of the world's most majestic mountains. After a lapse of many years, I make this the focus of all my visits to India.

With the start of World War II my father was posted to non-family stations and, as a result, we were left to be reared by my grandmother Najamai Bode, my mother's mother, who had no heart for this. She had borne three children. The first, Fali, died a teenager as a result of a brain injury when, as a spectator in a game of cricket, a ball hit his head. My mother, her oldest child, died at the age of thirty-three. My grandmother had no stomach for childrearing anymore and never filled the role of mother.

Grandmother looked and behaved like Queen Victoria. Her disgust and scorn for all things Indian was legendary. She refused to read the perfectly newsworthy *Times of India*, instead waited for the sea-mail copy of the *Daily Mirror*, six months out of date, to read all the local news, the murders, rapes and robberies in London. Her glass-covered cabinets were filled with volumes of Sir Walter Scott and Rudyard Kipling. Also Longfellow, Wordsworth and Tennyson. Walter Scott's *Ivanhoe* and what seemed to be interminable volumes of *Waverly* were safely kept under lock and key so neither she nor anyone else could get at them. They were books, but not for the reading. She had two season tickets to the fashionable Metro cinema for the 6.30 p.m. show on Sundays and always left the next seat vacant so that none of the proletariat could rub elbows with her. She wept copiously into her lacy lavender-scented handkerchiefs over the misfortunes of Betty Grable and Don Ameche but cared nothing for the three lost children in her charge.

The British left India in 1947 after a bloody and tumultuous partition of the country. I am not sure what the Parsis had expected, but there was a feeling of being monumentally jilted by them. They were now left to the mercies of an independent India, without the good offices of their British benefactors.

My grandmother continued her British life and was fueled by resentment against the locals whom she contemptuously called *dhotiadas*, referring to the *dhoti*, a white cotton garment draped from the waist that was worn by males. She was specially affronted when a hairy male leg was exposed. She blamed the *dhotiadases* for everything from the failure of the monsoons to the failure of the *Alphonso* mango crop.

My father retired in 1951 at the age of fifty-five, which was obligatory retirement age in the army, and although we looked at the possibility of moving to an independent apartment, this was not to be, and I started medical school continuing to live with my grandmother and now my father and sister Shirin in the fourth-floor apartment of 'Court View,' the first of a row of Art Deco apartment buildings opposite the Oval Green.

My first two years of basic sciences ended with multiple prizes and awards. To encourage female students they had separate awards for females, but had arrogantly not specified that prizes for males should be exclusive of females. The result was I won the female as well as the general prizes. I recently read that they had introduced a similar system for elected office in Rwanda. Separate female elections, but not having stipulated male-only elections, females stood in the male lines as well. As a result Rwanda is the only place in the world that has a female majority in the legislative section of the government.

In the third year of medical school we appeared for only one subject, Pharmacology. Pharmacology in my day was mainly learning by rote, and there was a particular student, the Pharmacology teacher's pet, who remembered all the doses and ingredients to the pills and medications we were presented with. To everyone's surprise she did not perform as expected, and an unknown called Amir Tejani won this award. Till this time I was peripherally aware of his existence, but now I had to take note. The day the results were announced I saw him in the pathology museum over a jar of cirrhotic liver. I said, 'Congratulations, Tejani,' and he smiled modestly and accepted my accolade.

Most thought him an upstart. His eight close male friends who had formed *bhailog*—a mafia-type brotherhood—were immensely elated, proving, they thought, that playing late-night poker while drinking bootleg liquor in prohibition-bound Bombay did no harm and, on the other hand, produced this star of Pharmacology. I saw it differently. I saw two shiny triangles below his eyes on his young cheeks that made him look as though he was always smiling.

Two clinical years later we graduated. Number16 won all the prizes and medals. All except Ophthalmology, which was awarded to the Chairman of Ophthalmology's son. Nepotism is a world-wide affliction.

At the University graduation ceremony, inexplicably, my father and sisters were not present, but when Number 16 collected all her awards there were loud cheers and whistles emanating from the Pharmacology star and his brotherhood. He walked me home across the Oval Green, and from then on we walked together.

I did six months of a surgical internship while Amir did pediatrics. I then went into six months of Obstetrics at a hospital that did 15,000 deliveries a year followed by a two-year Obstetrics and Gynecology registrarship. Amir obtained a diploma in Pediatrics and left for Africa during my registrarship to establish a practice and help his needy family. We wrote constantly.

So 1400 years ago his forebears had forced mine out of Persia. One would have hoped that these old insults would have been long forgotten. But no. Amir learned that there might be penalties for his parents if proper permission was not obtained for our marriage. He wrote an obsequious letter to the Aga Khan, the spiritual head of the Ismailis, to assure him that he would make every effort to convert me and that any children would be brought up as Ismailis. To placate my father he wrote a letter addressing him as 'Colonel Sir,' assuring him that any children would be brought up as Parsis and that I would be free to continue life as a Parsi. He may even have offered to convert himself. This seemed to placate everyone, and the wedding was set for December the first of 1959.

My sister Perrin came down to arrange things—I was oblivious to what went on since my registrar's job didn't end till the last week of November. Both sisters went to all the Parsi matrons to explain the marriage outside the community and were surprised at the enlightened response—these are modern times, they said. Privately, I think these pillars of the exclusive Parsi community felt—better you than me. We bought a resplendent silver and white silk sari, and the *darji* was called in to stitch dresses and sari blouses. Also a white nightie that Amir forever called night-whitie. That one and all the replicas that followed.

Amir arrived a week before the wedding. I learnt later that he had borrowed the airfare from Nurdin Walji, one of his more civilized drinking buddies, an extremely wealthy, quiet and generous person who never asked for the money back. Years later Nurdin gave Amir's father an accounting job, in spite of no formal qualification, in his high-flying Congo-based transport business.

Amir practically ran off the plane, wearing a cream-colored warm blazer in the humid Bombay winter, his one and only jacket. When I think of the times he raised eyebrows by wearing shorts at Christmas and to the most formal of functions, I think only purest love could have prompted a warm jacket in 80-degree weather. My father took Amir to Raab's, where Dad had his own suits stitched, and had a dark suit tailored for him. Amir continued that sweet tradition with his daughters' prospective husbands, and each had a splendid suit from Barney's in Manhattan when they were married. The ring totally flummoxed him, and the money for the diamond eternity ring that I am wearing as I write this was borrowed from my father. Also the fifteen rupees for the marriage license.

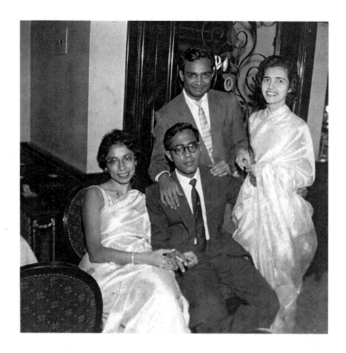

The wedding was to be a civil ceremony with the registrar coming to our spacious apartment. That apartment, much beautified and upgraded, now belongs to my younger sister Shirin. The ceremony was in the living room, and the formidable Parsi matrons—in full regalia of double rows of natural pearls, pendants and diamonds on their broad shelf-like breasts—sat around us. Amir stepped into the room and, surveying the ladies, took two steps back, then, with some determination, re-entered as the bejeweled breasts stared stonily at this upstart about to deflower Parsi womanhood.

The ceremony was quick and unromantic with some official phrases; however, the clerk absolutely insisted I give a ring to Amir. Panic—he had never and would never wear jewelry. Perrin tore off her own wedding ring, a flower-engraved gold ring, and gave it to me. I put it on his pinkie to satisfy the clerk. The ceremony over, Perrin grabbed it back. A particularly imposing and opera diva-type lady, a pillar of the community and a Justice of the Peace, took me aside and said she knew I was in love and all the rest of it, but to take one precaution: Keep a separate bank account. Today, long after his death, I still have a joint account.

There followed an alcohol-fueled reception in prohibition-Bombay and a dinner at Gaylord's Restaurant. Looking through old things preserved by Amir, I found the bill for this dinner. My father had paid fifteen hundred rupees, thirty-two dollars at the present rate of exchange, for a sumptuous dinner for a hundred guests.

Years later, in 1999, Amir and I were in Pune, India, to attend the wedding of my nephew Cyrus, Perrin's son, who was married on my birthday, November 21st. He too was marrying outside his Parsi community and had a civil ceremony but yearned for a religious blessing. So an enlightened Parsi priest came to Perrin's home and performed a mini version of the religious ceremony. In a religious Parsi wedding the couple sits on a flower-bedecked dais with parents and witnesses standing behind. Two or sometimes more Zoroastrian priests or 'Mobids' chant special wedding 'binding prayers'—very very long—while scattering rice on the couple with each promise and pronouncement. People who have endured this say you have to keep your eyes tightly shut to avoid getting the rice grains in your eyes. So couples have this rapt look on their faces when actually they are only avoiding the rice missiles.

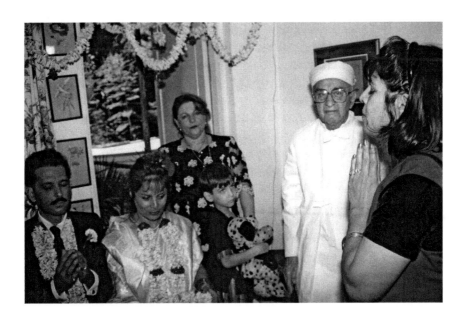

Cyrus, in his supreme elation over the blessing, wrung the hand of the priest and begged him to do the same for Amir and me, since we had never had this. The priest did, and the two of us held hands and sat with bowed heads in Perrin's small but gardened apartment and were remarried forty years after that day in 1959.

We spent the first month of our married life in a room at the Sea Green Hotel. Amazingly, years before, after my mother died and we moved to Bombay to live with my grandmother, I had attended a Montessori school at this same place—not a hotel till much later. The school was run by a Parsi woman who, no doubt, had talents unappreciated by me, but who pinched my cheeks to the point of acute pain as a greeting every morning.

The month was spent largely in the dismal immigration office, since my name change could only be effected after a marriage license was produced. I cannot remember any trauma with the overnight change from Bharucha to Tejani, and when I started life in Africa, people just knew me as Tejani. Certainly tidier than the path my daughters chose—Cena Tejani, mother of Tehmina and Shirin Pechefsky, and Sharyn Tejani, mother of Kiran and Amir Devine. Sharyn even threatened to have one of her sons use Tejani if the first name was Caucasian. That would give her sons different last names. Much tidier my way, if you can stand the loss. Typical of Rushna, my oldest daughter, she found middle ground and kept Tejani as a middle name.

We were to sail to Africa on the SS Karanja, a British-owned liner that sailed back and forth across the Indian Ocean from Bombay to Mombasa. A distant relative of mine—a cousin of my father's—was the ship's doctor and invited Dad on board for some iced German beer. Then, goodbye. Goodbye to that lone kindly figure, the man whose young wife died of typhoid fever when he was forty. I would see him only once again when I visited, very pregnant with my firstborn.

Our first stop was Karachi. I had won a pile of varied currency at Bingo and we spent indiscriminately. On boarding a bus heading to Clifton Beach I was shooed into the back caged enclosure with veiled women. We went to a movie theatre but balked when we realized that women sat separately from men. In the late evening we walked back to the docks, where the busy streets were still crowded, but entirely by males. Islam working its way through everyday life.

Then back to our cozy first-class cabin on the SS Karanja—a gift from my father. The rest of the passengers in the first class were all British. I wonder now at this group of expatriates traveling from one ex-colony to another soon-to-be ex-colony. They certainly did not seem to notice us—in their pursuit of whatever. And the Indians in the second and steerage classes stared at us as traitors. A miserable urinary tract infection was treated by the ship's doctor with three shots of Streptomycin, an antibiotic more toxic than effective, having caused hearing loss in thousands. My hearing today is magnificent in spite of this abuse.

There was a New Year's Eve party in mid ocean, and whistles and paper hats were donned by the adults around us. One sad-eyed inebriated English woman wrapped herself around a pole and said without the slightest smile, 'Whee, this is fun.' Clowns can be so sad.

We sailed into Mombasa—a confusion of light and rumbles of a never-before-visited continent—and Africa, no less. As I looked out, I romanticized... before me there were miles and miles of the unknown stretching out to the west. White adventurers who claimed to be discoverers—Africa was always there—Speke, Burton and Livingstone. *Simba* and *tembo*. Dineson and Hemingway. Best that I was unprepared for life with the passionate Tejanis. Best that I knew nothing about entering into the life of a minority and unloved community. Both these are more easily adjusted to in small slow doses.

Waiting quietly at the docks to receive us was Amir's cousin Mohamedali. A nod from him brought our luggage, another nod and it was carried to his waiting car. A short drive through the Indian section of this sweltering coastal town brought us to his home.

The apartment was on the second floor, living and dining room, two tiny bedrooms and a kitchen with wood and coal stoves. Mohamedali's family treated me with uneasy respect due, in their eyes, to my being a doctor, I guess. Matters were further complicated by my minimal knowledge of Gujerati, specially the pure Gujerati they used. The men spoke some English, but were not comfortable using it in the comfort of their home. A wonderful meal of several dishes was prepared, and the women made the *chapattis* as the men and I ate them. Me—not one of the women—having no idea of how a meal, much less *chapattis*, was created—and certainly not one of the men.

Come night, Mohamedali, his wife and two children, who all slept together in one room, gave their bedroom to us and slept on the floor in the living/dining room. Soon after we went to bed I saw a line of bedbugs emerge from the innards of the mattress. I told Amir I had seen a can of insecticide on the sideboard in the living room. Also on that sideboard was the family's entire collection of glassware. I warned him to get it noiselessly, for surely our complaint of bedbugs would offend if they woke. I heard him search around and then the most ear-splitting crash as the entire contents of the sideboard met the floor.

'*Mwizi, mwizi*'—'Thief, thief,' yelled Mohomedali armed with a stick. 'No, no,' said Amir—'I just need a glass of water,' returning to the bedroom without the water. Thus was I introduced to my spouse's lifelong state of klutz.

But much more than his bed, cousin gave me a gift. Hearing of my love for swimming and water, he would take us with a spicy packed lunch in his fishermen friends' boats to coves and grottos along the coast. They would stop at one of those pink and coral places, and we waded ashore. They then left and waited at some discreet distance while Amir and I ate and slept and swam. Years later, on return visits to Mombasa, I looked for those wild places, but they had vanished. I realize now that they must only have been accessible by sea and not by car.

We boarded the train to Kampala via Nairobi. Amir had promised me herds of wild life roaming the plains, and when I grew impatient, he pointed out dead trees saying, 'Ostrich! Giraffe!' He then and always could produce anything for my pleasure. When we went to the dining car to eat solid British-style gray meat and potatoes, unseen hands arranged the sleeping berths with fluffy whiter-than-white goose-down beddings. Even in the lonely depth of an upstate New York winter I have found goose-down asphyxiating—the thought of those plucked and molting feathers—but in that train speeding through the Kenyan lowlands it was home and romantic.

As the train slowed into Nairobi, I saw two familiar faces. The first belonged to my cousin JL. Years ago, he was in love and spurned by my sister Perrin, her maturity reflected in her reasons for the rejection—shorts too floppy, ears too flappy. He left Bombay and settled in Nairobi, and although never formally qualified as an architect, was commissioned to design cinemas and private houses. He married a young Kenyan-born Parsi woman from a wealthy, claustrophobic and exclusive family.

Also on the station was my childhood friend and distant cousin Perrin 'Honey' Mody. I had spent many an evening with her and her lovely and loving mother Sherubai to escape my grandmother. Honey was an air stewardess and flew the Bombay-Nairobi flight. These two smiling people from my past whisked us into a car for a quick tour of Nairobi National Game Park just outside the city. This was my first experience of the wild beauty and wealth of East Africa.

Lionesses at play, Thompson's gazelles on the wing, secretary birds criss-crossing the dirt roads. Elated and unbelieving, we boarded the train a couple of hours later for our eventual destination, Kampala, Uganda, my home for the next eleven years.

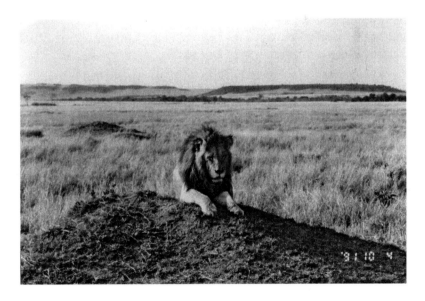

As we approached Kampala Station, I donned a demure outfit, a white-patterned purple silk sari, *chappals* and little make-up or jewelry—the picture of a modest Indian bride. I looked through the open railway carriage door at Kampala Station and saw a sea of people, all there to receive us. Very different from the lone father who saw us off at the Bombay harbor. As I focused, I realized that the women were dressed in fashionable Western-style high heels, masses of make-up and jewelry. My 'old country' dress, medium looks and glasses must have been a disappointment to these obviously appearance-conscious people. I found out later that the Aga Khan, the living spiritual leader of this Ismaili clan, had issued an edict that Western dress was to be adopted by all. Even older women who had worn a long dress and *pachhedi*, an ample scarf over their shoulders and head, all their lives, started wearing short dresses and all that went with them.

Worst of all, as I said, I had absolutely no understanding of the kind of Gujerati they spoke. Having lived the early part of my life at various postings with my army doctor father, my sisters and I learnt English as our first language. Later, during school, college and medical school in Bombay, I did learn some Gujerati, but it was a much-ridiculed Parsi version sounding like a heavy cockney accent to a BBC news reporter. And I had no knowledge of nuances or subtleties. If I had to use any, I would slip back into English. Their upper-class Gujerati and my cockney Gujerati cum English did not make a complementary beginning.

After a prolonged and confused arrival, we left for the family home in the Indian part of town. Number 8, Madras Gardens—just next to Bombay Gardens!

I had traveled thousands of miles and continents away and come from Bombay to Bombay Gardens!

Amir was the oldest of nine sibs. There had been ten in all. One, Khatoon, born after Amir, died in infancy, but the rest, five sisters and three brothers, have been our, and now my, friends through this long and restless journey. On that day early in January of 1960, they were all brought out to meet me. The youngest, Mohezin, his mother's pet, in a blue laced shirt. Mohezin's name was Amir's

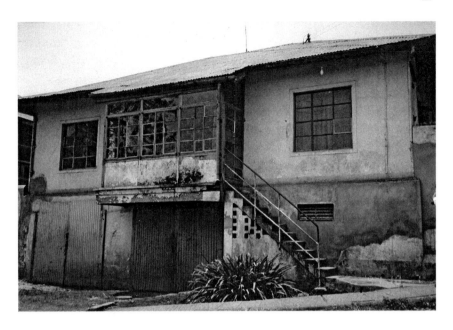

invention, from his much-admired Mohomedali Jinnah, the suave first prime minister of independent Pakistan. Firoze, handsome and lovable as he was then and always. Mary, shortened from Mehr-u-nissa, giving me every attention. Laila, deep in dysmennorrhoea but lovely to look at. Bahadur, already an intellectual, studying English literature at Makerere College. Through all the introductions I recognized him, Bahadur. Then, and over the years, he relieved me (in English) by allowing me to escape this earthy, funny, raucous family—into ideas and books.

Shamim, the youngest girl, had a double identity—her father called her Daulat, and her mother called her Shamim. Apparently they disagreed about her name at her birth, and just called her by their own choice of name. I learnt later that they had also disagreed about naming Amir, and he may have been named Sikander, which is the oriental name for Alexander (of Macedonia). Besides sounding somewhat absurd, this would have been even more unfortunate since it was Alexander of Macedonia who put a violent end to the great Zoroastrian emperor Darius, an event which led to the ultimate decimation of my ancestral Parsis in Persia.

Next in the family was Sultan, or Shahsultan as her father called her—quiet and withdrawn. The beauteous Gulshan was already married to another Amir and had a daughter, a year-old bonny dolly-jolly called Shilo.

And then there was that passionate mother. Our Ma, born and reared by a hated stepbrother on the coastal island of Lamu, she escaped her unhappy life by marrying this handsome fair tall young schoolteacher, Hadimohamed Tejani, in 1932 at the age of seventeen. They left Lamu in a *dhow* and were to live in Uganda, Tanzania, Kenya and Uganda again. Then followed the great flight to New York in 1972 as a result of Idi Amin's expulsion of all Asians, and in 1986, to the comfort and joys of family and community, to Vancouver, British Columbia.

Until a hysterectomy finally ended her distinguished obstetric career, Ma was either pregnant or breast-feeding for a great part of her life. She had her babies at home attended by a *Dai*, an Indian lay midwife, in Mengo, Sultanhamud, Kakamega and Singida. Her first, Amir, was born at Mengo Hospital, a missionary-run facility in Kampala. Once, many years later, I was visiting a patient at Mengo Hospital, and I asked to see the birth register for 1933. And there it was—in beautiful plump missionary script—'Born to Fatimabai Tejani on April 26th 1933, a boy weighing 7lbs.' And surprise! Amir had always claimed that all his faults and deficiencies could be attributed to a breech birth. He was born head first in the usual mundane manner. The upright rounded writing proved it.

I felt a quiet presence facilitating this first meeting. A tall fair handsome smiling man who after shaking my hand never addressed me directly. But he had an ear out for everything I said or even looked at. And quickly made it happen. This was Amir's father, Bapa, who treated me then and always with…the right word is *respect*. In Gujerati he always called me with formal *tame* rather than the familiar *tu*. His words and actions placed me on a high but comfortable pedestal.

Entebbe picnic

On the Sunday after we arrived we were to picnic at Entebbe, the seat of government in Uganda—about twenty miles from Kampala.

The day before, Saturday, Amir had taken me to the City Bar—a sort of initiation into his Saturday afternoons after morning consulting hours. Before I arrived on the scene he and his buddies would drink all Saturday afternoon and then eat a huge meal cooked by some long-suffering spouse or mother, sleep it off and then take in a movie at one of the four movie houses in town. Alas, his City Bar sessions were over. He introduced me to his friends, who were polite enough but clearly sad at my intrusion. We settled at a table under a canopy outside, and all were puzzled when I had no particular drink to call my own. Amir suggested I try a thing called 'Babycham'—a really sweet pseudo-champagne in a tiny bottle which I liked and drank whenever we went there.

A white woman came over and without so much as asking took a chair from our table. My paranoia caused me to mutter something to the effect that arrogance came with being white in the colonies. Amir laughed and introduced me to Nellie, the woman I had thought to be white. She was of mixed parentage—nusu-nusu—black and white—the most discriminated against in Ugandan society. I vowed to check, curtail, and rationalize my paranoia from then on.

The next day I had expected an early start for the picnic as we would have in Bombay to avoid the heat of the mid-day sun. But this was different. Perhaps people can be distinguished by the way they 'perform' their picnics. No thin cucumber sandwiches for this picnic. Ma, Mary, Laila and Sultan got themselves into the kitchen at 10 a.m. An elaborate meal of meat curry, rice and chapattis was to be prepared. Masses of onions were sliced fine and fried to a crisp, tomatoes and tumeric, cumin and chilli powder added. At the same time, the meat, which had been steeped in garlic and ginger, was bubbling slowly and the potatoes boiling in yet another pot. All were then assembled for a final tasting. As long as I can remember, Ma always tasted food by filling a spoonful, waiting for it to cool and then dipping her index finger in it for the smallest soupcon from which she was able to tell all it lacked.

Meanwhile, an assembly line had formed for the chapatti making. Ma had set the whole wheat dough to rest, Mary pulled out small balls and rolled them into perfect round thin flats and Laila baked them in a tava on a coal stove. One side just so, flip till it formed small blisters, and the last flip for a full puff. On to a waiting plate with Sultan ready to butter the top.

When cool enough, the saucepans were tied in large squares of cloth for stability and carried to the trunk of our Peugeot. Various other paraphernalia followed and finally, at about 1 p.m., we left, Amir driving, I and the two youngest sibs in the seat-beltless passenger seat and the remaining family in the back.

My first look at the countryside. Little homes with well-swept dirt front yards, each growing its own *matoke*—the green banana staple of Uganda—*cassava* and often some vegetables but always flowers—cannas, bougainvillea and all the year-round hedge-high poinsettias. A chicken or two clucking around, being fattened for a special occasion, and a goat tied to a post for an extra special event.

We arrived at the magnificent Entebbe Botanical Gardens and then began a prolonged discussion of possible picnic sites. I gathered that being next to water was essential. I later learnt that this was not to drink or play in, but to wash all the greasy dishes after we were done. The rivulet would soon turn to glistening tumeric and cumin gold.

We spread out our *makekas* and lolled till the food was reheated on the primus stove. After our soporific lunch we took the car to my first sighting of Lake Victoria, that mighty lake, the source of the

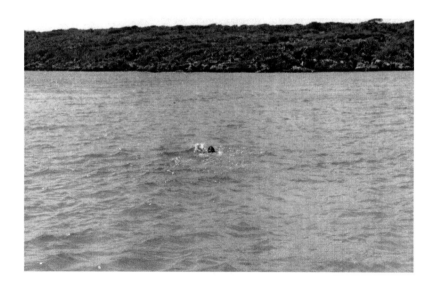

White Nile, a lake so large that the opposite bank was lost in mists and the curvature of the earth.

Unaware of the *schistosoma*—a parasite that plagued dwellers around the Nile and its sources—I plunged in and swam till I tired, much to Amir's anxiety. How many, many times he was to wait by the shore, all the world over, while I swam and swam. Lake Victoria was so huge with real waves that it was a surprise the water was sweet and not oceanic. Later, when we became conscious of *schistosomiasis*, my paranoia remembered that only Asians and a few blacks were swimming that day. The colonials obviously had some inside information.

Then back to the picnic site where real mixed sweet milky *chhai* was being prepared on the stove to be consumed with packets of 'Nice' biscuits. A slow and stately walk over the gorgeous gardens followed, so that we could work up an appetite for an impending evening meal. Clumps of spectacular ginger lilies stay in the memory. And then home again, home again.

Internal medicine — Mulago Hospital

But I could not abide staying at home in a household where I had not entered into its waves and rhythms. Where being married was strange enough—but also to be surrounded by a crowd who felt passionately about every little thing, and in a language I did not comprehend.

We had decided that I would work toward the MRCOG, the advanced degree in obstetrics and gynecology applicable in Britain and the colonies. On enquiry at Mulago Hospital, the teaching hospital of the Makerere Medical School, I was told there were three training positions to be created from September of that year, with the objective of grooming candidates for the MRCOG. I applied and was accepted for one of them. The requirements for MRCOG also included six months of internal medicine. I learnt that there was indeed a position in internal medicine, but no salary line. I could do it without remuneration. Weighing the situation, I needed the six months of internal medicine, and, above all, I had to be out of that house during the day. I never gave any thought to what had to be an important issue—we needed the money to repay past debts, pay for the newly acquired home and the running of a household of many. It had to have been a heavy thought with Amir, but he never burdened me with any obligation to earn a living.

So I took this moneyless job as house physician in internal medicine. The senior consultant in my team was the crabby beetle-browed Dr. G, who seemed to take an instantaneous dislike to me. He had the typical stereotypic opinion of Indians and often, in my presence, referred to them as *dukawallas*—a derogatory term meaning shopkeepers—more like shopkeepers who could never rise above the daily grind of bringing in the shillings and not above twisting the truth to do it. I initially appreciated Dr. G's knowledge of Luganda, the language of the Muganda tribe, most populous in the Kampala area. Later I realized that he always asked the same initial question and followed it with the same backups, irrespective of the patients' answers.

It was learning by being plunged into the midst of totally unfamiliar situations and clawing out, errors and all—with Dr. G maliciously watching. His first assistant was J, a South African of Indian origin. I later came to know that J was an intelligent and a good doctor; however, in the poisoned atmosphere where we met, I do not remember any learning or guidance coming from him. All I remember was his acquiescence in all that Lord G proclaimed. No doubt a tainted memory.

J once sat next to me at a dinner given by the local doctors. He was invited as a respected consultant and I as a spouse. I was wearing my mother's engagement ring, an uncut emerald with an orca-like flaw in it. Since it lacked the facets and flash of a modern cut emerald, most people thought it was a glass bead. I saw him stare at it, and before long it was in his hands, him stroking it, all the while talking of the beauty and science of gems, of which I was quite ignorant. It was the only time I saw passion in him. Decades later he was 'diasporaed' to Western Australia, but while in the U.S. he called me about a 'light' article he had read written by me in the *Lancet* on guinea worms and gentle hands. Even forty years later, I recognized his voice immediately—South African/British with a hesitancy all his own. He scolded me for not knowing the difference between Buganda, the province; Baganda, the people; Muganda, a person; Luganda, the language; and Uganda, our country. I remembered how he always obsessed on detail while I, having to expedite my learning, often muddled things of this sort.

I was completely unfamiliar with tropical diseases, exotic sexually transmitted diseases. The local malignancies such as Kaposi sarcoma and Burkitt's lymphoma and primary liver malignancies were common at that time before the advent of AIDS and resulted in the development of a solid tumor center for clinical management and research. I had never even heard of endomyocardial fibrosis, the common and most deadly heart affliction of the area, where the heart is reduced to a fibrotic mass with tiny chambers unable to accommodate or pump. I had to work many times harder than others just to stay afloat, with Cecil Loeb as my constant companion and guide.

Nsenene nights

Nothing annoyed Dr. G as much as a ward brimming full of patients. The night after I had been on call it was always bursting at the seams because I lacked discrimination and judgment in admitting patients and, fearing the worst, I would admit them all. Dr. G would avoid the wards the morning after I had worked till J had cleared the decks for him. The mornings after *nsenene*—grasshopper—nights were a total disaster as I admitted all the drunks for fear of what might happen if I let them wander or drive the streets.

One man was admitted about once a week for acute alcoholic intoxication. Instead of being subject to recriminations, he was the ward favorite, the pet joker who was fondly tolerated, treated with rest, hydration, sedation and then let loose with no further direction. He was what he was. No Betty Ford rehab for him. Slim and smiling, he was confident in his expectation to be tolerated. He was a particular favorite of Dr. G's—a child forever—exactly how G wanted him.

If his liver was damaged, there was no clinical evidence of it. His drink was home brew—deadly *waragi* made from fermented bananas and grain in an evil never-washed metal pot over a wood-burning stove set up in a clearing in the *charo* that belonged to him and his cronies. No women and children allowed.

As he recovered I asked him how much he had drunk this time.

I over-stepped. By tacit consent, no one was allowed to ask those questions. His smiling face became stony, and he turned away to the next patient and started a conversation in Luganda to pointedly exclude me. My righteousness had no place in his life. No help for me from colleagues or consultants. Let him be.

On certain African nights when there had been the correct duration of dry weather followed by the right amount of rain, the grasshopper-like insects called *nsenene* came visiting our town. The aroma of relief to the parched red Kampala earth rescued by warm rains—something to remember forever.

On these warm soft nights clouds of *nsenene* entered the town, flocking in great droves beneath the streetlights. A wild *nsenene* night. The locals left all business and with white bedsheets, food and drink, camped under the streetlights for the night. Occupation of the area under the light by one group gave squatter's rights, and others could not join and compete.

With much talk, discussion and laughter, four women held the corners of the white sheets and shook them. The men lounged and drank. The *nsenene* were irresistibly attracted to white and made suicidal charges into the sheet. When a big enough haul was completed, the corners of the sheet were brought together and the bundle emptied into large Nubian narrow-mouthed woven baskets to prevent escape. Meanwhile, an open charcoal stove and pan were fired and the *nsenene* readied for roasting. It needed a delicate touch and much experience to hold each one and pluck the wings and head off without tightening one's hold, which would result in squashed *nsenene*. Squashed *nsenene* were discarded and never eaten.

The insects were now incapacitated and could not escape. The wings were inedible anyway. A few minutes on the hot coals turned them into tasty crispy morsels that added to the feast. The groups ate and drank the night away, and the remaining roasted *nsenene* appeared at the market the next day. They sold at a few cents for a quarter pound packed tightly into newspaper cones. I often bought them, although there were no takers, other than myself, at my home. Tasted like a cross between crisp french fries and shrimp. A little ketchup—delicious. And their wingless headless plight made them less recognizable as insect fare.

Drunken *nsenene* nights produced much traffic at the Emergency Room and in the hospital. The police were tolerant and even participated. The routine went something like this. If someone became loud and intolerable, he or she was reported to the often-carousing police. They were charged with being drunk and disorderly and carted off to the home of a police surgeon. My spouse was one of these, and I often watched as 'tests' were applied. Walk on an impossibly straight line. Repeat 'Red lorry, yellow lorry' ten times. I later discovered that it was a Bantu thing to say 'R' for 'L.' 'Prum' pudding instead of 'plum' pudding. No one passed this deadly test. As far as I recall, no objectivity was added in the form of tests for breath or blood alcohol levels.

It was after such a sumptuous night that I walked into the early morning ward certain to see our favorite patient there. *Nsenene* nights were more legitimate than just drunken nights, and he would have taken full advantage of their legitimacy. Where was he?

He had been admitted comatose in the early hours of the morning. He was treated as usual, but this time he had come to say goodbye. He slipped away a few hours later. We comforted ourselves saying that he went out doing what he did best.

Gentle hands

We worked in teams. 'Firms,' we called them. Dr. G gave me such negative times that I jumped at the opportunity to join Professor Williams when a vacancy occurred on his team. Prof. Arthur Williams was the Chairman of Internal Medicine at Makerere Medical School and Mulago Hospital. My hopes that this would be a regular teaching and healing experience were not disappointed, and the next few months were busy and full of an academic kind of fun.

Professor Williams had two first assistants: Dr. Gerry Shaper, a brilliant young physician from South Africa, willing to teach and explain and help whenever I and others needed assistance, and Dr. George Monekoso, a somewhat sardonic but extremely knowledgable internist from Nigeria. And suddenly the seduction of an academic life became apparent. Slow, deliberate professorial rounds with civilized appraisals inclusive of all levels of roundees and specially inclusive of, and considerate and respectful of, the central point—the patient. Over the years, I realized again and again that major and memorable teaching and learning occurred at the bedside. 'Contemplative rounds,' Lewis Thomas called those intense times.

But I had to earn my place on that distinguished team.

An early pregnancy with its associated miserable nausea intruded on this idyll. I thought I knew what I was doing with my professional life—internal medicine, a year of Ob/Gyn and then some time in London to appear for the MRCOG board examination. How this pregnancy that had occurred with no real planning was going to allow all this, I, we, had not figured out. I smile when I hear residents today somewhat mockingly speak of an 'unplanned pregnancy.' Like mine so many tears and years ago.

In my first week with Prof. Williams I was tested for my mettle. The newest house officer—me—was given the case. Experience, knowledge, technical skills were not an issue. The assignment would have been the same in any medical hierarchy, even outside the 'Oh, so British' colonies. This case was perceived as a mindless arduous task.

The patient was a regular. He walked into the hospital with no appointment or prior call. He followed no protocol. He did not triage through clinic or Emergency Room which were the entry points for other patients. Nurses knew he approached by the 'tap tap' of his cane—not white, just a much-used gnarled branch from a hardwood tree. He turned, found a chair and sat. No words needed.

Greeting *sebo*, greetings *nyebo*. How are your *matoke* fields, your goats, your cows, your family? All was well. I watched the easy relaxed scene between patient and nurse. Was I ever going to have the confidence and ease to enter into it?

Even at a distance I saw he was covered with white blisters. What?

Dr. T, you've heard of guinea worms? Guinea worms! Every cranny on his extremities was infested. Sparser elsewhere. On his palms and soles, one milky lesion flew into another. Is there an anthelmenthic for this? Yes, a grin, you.

My instructions: Antiseptic. Abrade the skin to expose the beast. Scoop it out. Do not draw blood. Identify the head as proof of a complete job. Above all, do not break off this longest of worms afflicting humans. Dire pictures of energized re-growth were threatened if breakage was committed. If there was stubborn resistance, roll it on a Q-tip and let it dangle. More antiseptic. On to the next one. My early pregnancy reminded me of its presence by a wave of nausea. Somebody brought needles, iodine, gauze.

I walked over and spoke a greeting in English to this man who spoke only *Luganda*. He did not even bother to turn his trachoma-clouded eyes to me. Almost contemptuous. 'Yet another novice,' he seemed to say to himself.

Gloved, bent over, I started on the first lesion. Picked it with a hypodermic needle and watched the rolling coils tumble out. Applied pressure to the sides with my thumb and index finger and swept the cavity, its cozy shelter, with the sides of a needle. Identified the head of the monster. Did it five more times. More nausea.

I drew up a chair. This was a good move. I perceived a change. He turned to me briefly. A system. I needed a system. Across the palm, back and forth, back and forth till done. Would this tire him? What did he want? Ask him, nurse.

'Do what suits you.' In a life-and-death ward, my question was inconsequential.

Imperceptibly, a rhythm developed. I had always derived perverse pleasure from squeezing blackheads. Here was what I always wanted to do to unwilling sisters and spouse, only on a much grander scale. However, most of the pleasure in the blackhead thing was the howling dissent of the victim. This man neither protested or assented.

Both hands and soles were done. The few that refused to leave their nests were left rolled on dangling sticks. He had to sleep now, I was told. I was dismissed.

I returned the next morning. Would he be there? Yes, sitting on the same chair as though he had never moved. But he acknowledged my footstep. I sat.

A nurse said, 'He is Moslem. His name is Ishmael.'

He echoed, 'Ishmael, *mishkini*' — Ishmael, the beggar.

Ishmael, what seas have you sailed before you were trapped by trachoma?

I began again, and a comfort started growing in our relationship.

What was this all about? Brilliant diagnosis? Technical triumph? Or just care-giver with bowed head and the timeless patient?

Most lesions were cleared by evening. He had a faintly girlish look about him because of the dangling white wormy rolls on Q-tips, like braids on a sweet girl. He ate and slept. I left.

The chair was empty the next day.

Months later I receive a gift. Tap, tap. Enter Ishmael. He asks, *'Ari wa mpola ngando?'* — 'Is gentle hands still here?'

Wastage

My pregnancy was associated with annoying nausea but worse, for the first—and last—time in my life, I could not get to sleep. The constant calls from the ward further destroyed my night. One night at 1 a.m. I had a call to attend a patient who had a seizure. Amir said he would go instead of me. 'Aren't I Dr. Tejani?' I gratefully went back to restless tossing and turning; however, the next morning I was appropriately admonished for my deception by my consultant Gerry Shaper. Instead of slinking unobtrusively in and out, Amir had drawn maximum attention to himself by parking outside a hospital fence and vaulting the fence to save himself the walk up and down Mulago Hill. He then made sure that all the nurses assisted him, laughed and talked to him, all the time insisting that he was Dr. Tejani. One of them apparently noticed his sex and ratted.

Thalidomide was my companion during those nauseous, sleepless months. I found that it suppressed my nausea, helped me to sleep, and yet I could wake to attend to a call, drive and go right back to sleep. It was really not as awful as it sounds. Truly a wonder drug. I was completely unconscious of that 42nd day when it cast its spell on the tiny developing limb buds. It is hard to accept that a sensitive mother could not feel this tragedy occurring.

Time passed, and I was twelve weeks pregnant. The nausea had disappeared, and I organized weekend escapes to explore the White Nile—meeting it at different spots as it arose from Lake Victoria in Jinja and meandered, rushed and swirled to its meeting in Khartoum with the Blue Nile that originated in Lake Tanu in the Ethiopian mountains.

On one occasion we drove through a butterfly-dense dirt road headed to the Bujagali Falls. The butterflies were so thick that the windshield of the car was causing slaughter. We stopped and stood outside the car to watch as they came and settled on us with a touch like quickening, the initial flickerings of a tiny fetus. Covered in butterflies and smiling were we. Whenever a pregnant woman asks me what fetal movements feel like, I always say 'like a butterfly.'

At the falls and rapids we played the day away. Toward afternoon, the most precarious but bold swimmer Amir descended into the rapids and sang a tuneless song to prove he was not afraid. 'Ram-pam-po,' it went, and at the third 'ram-pam...,' it faded as he got caught in the current and swirled away. This was the first of two times I saved him from a watery fate. I hurried over slippery rocks to a swirly pool where the current had transported him, plunged in and pressed him against a rock till a calm moment and then we swam back to a shallow point where other arms pulled us out. The second was decades later in 1984 on a trip to Galapagos, snorkeling in the icy waters of a sunken volcano in the company of ballerina seals—so clumsy and flat-footed on land, but sleek and fleet as they made rings around us in the water. The nature guide warned a trillion times to swim out against the current so that the current could float you back when you were tired. Amir let the current carry him out. I kept my eye on him while I was doing it right, and sure enough I saw him struggling back, having thrown off his mask and snorkel. I went out to him and we battled the current coming back together.

As we gathered up to leave Bujagali Falls, a long slim-waisted wasp circled and stung me on the calf. I became light-headed and nauseous and had some difficulty breathing. Amir always kept his battered doctor's bag with him—I still have it—and miraculously was able to give me a shot of adrenaline within minutes of the sting. A fair exchange for the drowning I had saved him from less than an hour before.

Waves of itchy skin rashes followed in the next days. At sixteen weeks the obstetrician announced no growth from the twelve-week visit. A few days later, a bewildering painful loss at Nakasero Hospital which was replete with formidable Matron, disciplining sisters and no visiting. No help for breaking hearts—no help.

'No point in showing her this hopeless fetus.' Get over it.

Trembling Amir told me it was a boy. Would have been middle-aged today. I never quite finished with him. I feel as though I abandoned him by my weak agreement not to look and think goodbye. As life went on, I had my quota of three powerful girls and never thought about the absence of a son, till decades later we had grandsons. And I first missed a son when I saw Amir playing ball interminably with our oldest grandson Ellis.

The story of thalidomide evolved. Exquisitely timed 42nd-day exposure resulted in this fatal marriage with developing limbs. A doctor friend's daughter was born with little flappy limbs. A positive attitude allowed applause for all of life's regular milestones. A few nights ago, I watched a concert from Lincoln Center. Beverly Sills interviewed the bass baritone, who was shortly to perform. He was gracious, eloquent, unassuming, balding and in his forties. But then I saw him walk onto the stage. Less than four feet tall, perfectly formed head — which had been interviewed earlier — and little flipper limbs. And that deep golden voice. His mother must have been swallowing thalidomide on the same nights that I did.

I cannot unravel luck from loss. Thalidomide and wasp sting had to be a rare combined insult. I and others call this fetal wastage. A sad waste. A waste with our love and kisses. We donate our healthy children to the public domain, to take their place in life. But this one remains forever private.

A short recovery and a drive to the game park in Nairobi to forget and heal. I watched those lionesses at ease with cubs in fearsome play. A cheetah with absurd furry young. Vultures waiting their turn at a wildebeast kill. A spotted hyena slinking and skulking. A crystal moment as we were leaving the park — a group of delicate Thompson's gazelles in a sun-dappled lea suddenly lifted their heads in unison, up and to the right at some invisible danger. It helped.

After that, I lived my life thinking a wasp sting would be fatal. At first I carried epinephrine, but over the years, since I never met a wasp, I lost the syringe that I carried around in my pocketbook. One evening more than thirty years after my initial wasp encounter, I put my hand into the heart of a clump of sorrel in my kitchen garden in Ossining, New York. I felt a sharp sting as I withdrew my hand. A deadly slim-waisted wasp flew out. I sat down on the dirt surrounded by peas and spinach waiting for the inevitable. Nothing happened. African and American wasps are races apart.

Common sense prevailed after this first pregnancy. There would be no more till I had completed my MRCOG board examinations.

Going back to work after the few days I had taken off for the pregnancy loss and game park was horrendously difficult. What did I fear? I went into the ward through a side door. Without lifting my head so as to meet anyone's eyes, I picked up the charts for my side of the ward and started work. I had just started feeling that splendid euphoric pregnant feeling that the end of nausea brings. That feeling of superiority over all males and non-pregnant females. That genetic empowerment. May not win the Nobel, but will leave my genetic traces forever. And now climb down.

My civil and civilized colleagues did not fail me. Those who did not know did not know. Those who did murmured sympathy and then just got on with business.

I hear a song in my head

Twice a week, I saw patients at all-day clinics. These were walk-in arrangements and whoever came was eventually seen.

A young man with shiny skin of dark black and midnight blue came to the clinic alone. A blue-black skin illuminated from within. Doe-brown almond eyes with embroidered lashes. His face spoke to his ancient Nilotic origin.

He waited his turn on a rickety chair in the clinic. Women seated nearby greeted him, but he did not return their familiarities. No smile for these bustly, busty women in their Victorian style *basutis* and striped under-cloths. Patients arriving after him jostled their way to attention while he sat waiting and listening, too young for the whittled cane he held between his legs.

Hey, come on, if you want *dagara*—medicine—today. Some physical prodding before he wavered to his feet to sit before me. A conversation with the translator lasted too long. I helplessly distrusted these translator sessions which yielded monosyllables after minutes of animated discussion.

I intervened in the prolonged exchange that had now entered into argument. Through the open window of the barracks-like clinic, I saw my ride arriving. One car had to serve the needs of all the working people in the large family. I needed to get out of the clinic. Others were waiting to be picked up and taken home.

'What does he say?'

'He is *wazimu*—crazy.'

What must the patient think? An argument instead of the ancient art of medical history-taking and then a diagnosis of insanity. At my insistence, pleading almost, I was told that this *wazimu* says he hears a song in his head. Anything else? He walked here alone from his village because he hears a song in his head.

The insistent ride was still outside the window. My patient lay down to be examined. I went over his head, eyes, ears, nose and throat. His heart, his lungs, his abdomen. His extremities. His cranial nerves, his motor and sensory nervous systems.

'Tell him I do not find any problem.'

Vindicated and victorious, the translator relayed the message.

'But,' said the patient, 'you did not listen to my head.'

He pulled the chest piece of the stethoscope to his head. Feeling foolish, I donned the ear-pieces.

A wailing desert song, like the *hamsin* desert winds that blow for fifty days and nights with dust and sand obscuring the world. It ebbed and blew, ebbed and blew. He saw that I saw. He lived with a song in his head. Others live with fear, anxiety, ambition. He lived with a song.

I admitted him to the wards. I was always taught to have a plan. What plan could I have when I was clueless? The next day troops of house officers and medical students surrounded him, listened and discussed him over his quiet presence in the arrogant way that comes naturally to us. A touching moment always when he grasped the stethoscope and guided it to the wildest windiest spots in his head.

Professor Williams (this was before the great age of imaging) applied the only imaging we had. An astonishing X-ray picture. The inside of the skull had indentations like beaten silver. Or, if you change your perspective from negative to print, a Medusa effect, skull deficiencies filled with writhing snakes.

Our Professor did not take long to figure arterio-venous malformation. A communication between an artery and vein in the brain resulted in elevated arterial pressures flowing into thin-walled veins, causing them to puff and writhe and sing in agony.

The patient's mood was celebratory. He was right instead of crazy. There was a music-maker in his head.

What next? Even today, forty years later, some arterio-venous malformations are best left untouched if abutting or involving significant parts of the brain. A surgical 'cure' could be more disabling than the disease. Every so often, a patient would be flown from our African plains to the hallowed halls of a London teaching hospital for a miracle cure. Much fanfare was attached to this act of grace. Unfortunately, these cases had to be forgone successes. No failure or error was allowed. The song man's vessels were everywhere, endangering all that he retained. Too risky—he did not qualify.

A diagnosis was made. There was nothing to be done. The prognosis: unpredictable bleeding from the thin-walled snaky monsters with expectations of disability and sudden death.

I mumbled my regrets.

'But,' he consoled me, 'it does make a change in my life.' The specialists at the teaching hospital had agreed there was a song. He had not really expected the song to be silenced. With dignity and humor, he said he might even miss it if it went away.

We were graceful in those days in allowing patients to stay in hospital till they were ready to leave. He contemplated for a few days and one morning was gone.

A nurse who whispered her goodbyes said he was smiling when he left.

The smallpox village

At the start of the Internal Medicine rotation, all the new doctors were required to be vaccinated against smallpox as we eventually were required to rotate through the 'village.' My turn came about three months into my rotation.

It was a trek through the woodlands. You left the barracks-like ward of the main hospital and walked down a dirt road—the bright red earth of Uganda. You approached a clearing—a sylvan setting—and started to hear voices. I was told that once a case occurred, the entire family was brought here to isolate them from the rest of the community.

A tiny settlement appeared with a few one-room cottages and a common outhouse. Outdoor wood fires with families cooking and living. A peaceful scene with a woman steaming *matoke* in banana fronds, filling the air with its starch banana smell. Children had marked out a hopscotch plane—the same as they do the world over—and one slender girl cast her pebble in the first square and did the universal hop...one, one, one, two, one, two, turn, and back again, lifting the pebble on the way back.

I greeted the woman who was preparing the meal for the families who accompanied the two adult male patients. Had she been vaccinated? Yes, and the children. She stirred a pot with the aroma of peanuts—a sauce to go with the *matoke*. The soft comfort of small things.

But this was no small thing. I parted the soiled curtains that led to the single room in the cottage. A man lay quietly on a battered bed with eyes shut, unsleeping. He had contacted an infected person four weeks ago and had this rash for a week. The smallpox rash is different from chicken pox—and deadly. It starts on the torso and spreads peripherally. All the lesions are in the same stage of development unlike the waves of lesions at different stages with chicken pox. And patients are febrile, toxic and deathly sick.

The lesions covered every spot on him, often running one into the other. They were raised into fluid and blood-filled blisters with hemorrhages dotting the skin between them. A mild nod to isolation—there was a battered stethoscope hanging on a rusty hook in each of the cottages. I checked his lungs for pneumonia, not happy about using the same earpieces that must have been used by crowds of previous caregivers. I never understood how normally fastidious people seem to share stethoscopes without a problem. Think of the innards of the wax and dirt-encrusted ears one has encountered. And yet, even today, 'Can I borrow your stethoscope?' is a request that cannot be turned down.

Maddening irritation of the rash was reduced by the family applying slaths of calamine lotion which appeared to be the one commodity we had masses of. Rose pink caked the crevices of the jagged sores. How will it ever wash off? More ominous, it may never need to be removed.

And then we waited. Some went on to an untreatable state with inability to clot, confluent hemorrhages, bleeding to death from multiple sites. Some developed irrevocable pneumonia. And some passed it on to other family members who ruefully crept into bed with the original patient. Some recovered, but were marked forever by scars that covered the face and the rest of the body like a rugged Mars-scape. My patient did recover, scarred and weak, but not before his daughter, the hopscotch girl, had to lie down with him covered in a lesser rash. Timely vaccination attenuated the attack.

Thank you, milkmaids. Thank you, Edward Jenner, for taking notice of the minor cow-pox milkmaids developed in lieu of deadly smallpox. The brilliant concept of cross-immunity. Vaccination became a religious rite, and health-care workers criss-crossing the remotest corners of the world have told us we have triumphed and smallpox is no more.

We slept our happy sleeps for years till now we read of this ancient virus being used as a weapon, more deadly than anthrax since it spreads aerially without direct contact. Spreads through unseen droplets.

And an unvaccinated population! Don't want to hear any more of that story.

A little love nest

After six months of living with Tejanis young and old, passionate, funny, giving, taking, I needed a quiet space.

Two domestic accidents lent urgency to my need to leave. I had the need to somehow prove some culinary ability. The reason for this was difficult to explain, but I felt that it was the only language I could talk to them in. I tried my hand at a few things but I lacked any grounding in the principles. I kept writing my father to send recipes—my father who had never set foot in a kitchen. Finally he sent me the Parsi bible—the 'Time and Talents' cookbook put together by the formidable Parsi matrons who had daunted Amir at our wedding. Each page of the book is footnoted with a quotation illustrating the Parsis' obsession with all things British and European. The quotes varied from sweet, 'I will make my kitchen, And you shall keep your room, Where white flows the river, And bright blows the broom' —to chauvinistic, 'A man is in general better pleased when he has a good dinner upon his table, than when his wife talks Greek'—to exotic, 'Prunes of Bokhara, and sweet nuts from the far groves of Samarcand,'—to French, 'Dit moi ce que tu mange, je dirai qui tu est.' And a good Parsi thought, 'Papri ma gos, te to maru dost'—'Broad beans cooked with meat are my friend.'

I set out to make 'A hundred almonds chicken curry.' The family indulged me somewhat mockingly. But Bapa (Amir's father) went out shopping with his cloth bag. He bought the fresh chicken, mercifully killed, plucked and cut into pieces, counted out the hundred almonds at the 'ration' store, bought two coconuts which left me clueless till someone cracked them, scooped out the meat, poured hot water on them and squeezed out the coconut-flavored water. I was then given a deep pot to minimize spills and mess.

The first instruction was to measure out one and one-half pounds of *ghee*, clarified butter. One and one half pounds! I still have the book to prove my innocence, but I did not figure the misprint at the time. The next edition apologized and said one and one-half tablespoons. Anyway, in went the huge amount of *ghee*. The onions and tomatoes disappeared in the sea of grease followed by the drowning chicken, the carefully counted pounded almonds from which further oil seeped, and the coconut milk, also fat-filled. I thought maybe with the spices and potatoes the grease would disappear and the edibles would emerge. But no such thing happened. By now I had an interested audience. Also a hungry one. One more look at the fatty mess and I felt the blood rush to and then away from my head and I passed out. When I woke up the chicken had been retrieved and turned into a delicious creation by these consummate family cooks.

My second cooking fiasco was during my pregnancy. I had a yen to eat *bhinda*—okra—once more misguidedly insisting that I make them. Once again Bapa whipped out his cloth bag and went to the market and came back with the best fresh green baby *bhinda*. I was warned many times not to—repeat *not* to—allow even a drop of water into the cooking. Ignoring this I washed them, leaving the water drops clinging, and then added water while they were cooking. In a few minutes, a transformation occurred. From fresh bright green they turned into a mucinous mass. Long slimy threads criss-crossed the pot worse than a bad cold or the worst cervicitis. On lifting a spoonful the stringy *spinbarkeit*, the mucous strings I could draw it out into, were a foot long. The familiar blood to and away from the head recurred and I was out again. This time there was no retrieval and even the alley cat that came begging every evening was spared this horror.

I have passed out only three times in my life. The first time was before these two cooking mishaps. I had just graduated from basic sciences in medical school, and a resident thought he would give me a treat by allowing me into the delivery room. The room was overheated and I can still see the agonized woman pushing against her bulging perineum while two midwives talked and laughed over her. I was soon flat on the floor and missed the delivery. When I opened my eyes even the patient was peering over the bed and laughing at me.

Although we could hardly afford two residences, Amir struggling to pay the bills and debts and me doing unpaid work, we found and moved into a small, newly built third-floor apartment in the town on Salisbury Road. We rented from a family who ran a car dealership on the main floor. The son who ran the store was a pleasant heavyset person with a violent limp, the result of an old attack of polio. We were walking distance from the stores and from my favorite store in Kampala, a used bookstore called Haideri Book Mart that sold marvelous old books for the equivalent of a few cents. I still have a cookbook that I bought from Haideri's for a couple of shillings entitled 'With a Jug of Wine.' Not exactly the 'basics' cookbook I needed, but I soon discovered that even the worst swill improved with a cupful of wine.

Periodically Haideri's would hold Persian rug auctions, and I still possess a Qum weave bought for the equivalent of seventy-five dollars. Years later I saw a match to it in Manhattan being sold for thousands of dollars. Qum later assumed significance as the home of the original Ayatollah, the Ayatollah Khomeini. The carpet is typical of that village, squares with flowery motifs in each square. One always represented the tree of life.

You entered this little blue heaven from a back walkway, huffing and puffing to the third floor as there was no elevator. We used the hallway as a dining room, complete with formica dining table and chairs covered in rexine—a shiny synthetic faux leather. This was not because of our concern for the dwindling forests, but a fad of the time. This room led to two rooms, both floored in that elegant zig-zag herringbone parquet so typical of Uganda. A carpenter finally made a double bed for us, and for the first time we did not have to fight the *kappa*, the space between pulled-together twin beds. A large sky-blue kitchen with blue counters and blue bookshelves completed this lovely, loving and love-filled tiny home.

A typical day would start with letting in the houseboy—called simply *mtoto*, child—and the newspaper, the *Uganda Argus*. *Mtoto* would make sweet milky *chai*, and we would awaken, shower and drive to Amir's practice opposite the Ismaili mosque, which had already been opened by Husseini, Amir's assistant and our driver and general helper. Young handsome gentle Husseini was a converted Ismaili. I heard that such conversions of local people occurred with the lure of new clothing. Husseini was indeed excellently dressed. This and all mornings Husseini was dressed in a white-than-white open-necked shirt tightly buttoned over his naturally muscular pectorals and short sleeves to display his steroid-unassisted biceps. I often looked at him and thought how magnificent he would look in a traditional African kanzu, a long flowing white robe, and a gold-embroidered red velvet *topi* on his head. Or even the wilder flowing flamboyant leopard skins and bark cloth of pre-British times. I never asked him whether he ever wore traditional clothing in his real life.

Amir would start his morning work, and Husseini would drive me to 8 Madras Gardens, where the working crew would join me. I would then be dropped at Mulago Hospital and Mary and Laila at the telephone exchange where they worked. At midday we would reverse the route and all assemble at Ma's home for a fast but huge meal. And then back to work with Husseini doing the driving. In the evening Husseini would pick us all up from work and take us home. We would leave him at the practice to make his own way to wherever, and Amir and I would drive home. With my irregular times inconveniencing all, it became clear that I would need driving instruction. We did not bother with the next step, another car, as it was beyond our non-existent budget. Amir took me to the parade grounds at lower Kololo Terrace and with much frustration, derisive laughter and raw anger, I learnt how to drive. I eventually got to be much the better driver. Nonetheless, I always had the highest insurance premiums because of accidents. Other motorists just stayed away from Amir's fast unpredictable ways, and he seemed never to be involved in accidents.

The dependence on houseboys was astounding. If *mtoto* did not turn up one day, there would be confusion and near desperation. I would leave him instructions as to what to keep ready for the evening meal and then prepare it with open recipe book propped. I was quick to realize that cooking was common sense mixed with flexibility. If the crab cakes disintegrated, they could be converted into crab scrambled eggs.

Our immediate neighbors, just a thin wall away, were a Scottish couple who played the Beatles all day long. 'A Hard Day's Night' became our signature homecoming tune. As each evening progressed, the Beatles gave way to bitter high-volume quarreling. One could only imagine the Scottish couple consuming Scotch and proceeding with the evening's recriminations. Then suddenly silence—we pictured the comatose couple on the floor. The next morning it was back to the Beatles.

Katikiro

Old Uganda was divided into four kingdoms with melodic names, but harsh realities—Buganda, Busoga, Toro, and Ankole. Of them the power lay with King Freddie, the Kabaka of Buganda, the King of the Baganda people, educated, professional, a force for future governance.

The Kabaka's affairs were managed by the golden-tongued Katikiro, his prime minister. The Kabaka was worshipped and bowed to. No human was allowed to stand taller. His minions shuffled along on their knees to meet this requirement. Such adulation was a passport to living in a world removed. The Katikiro twisted and turned affairs of state and maintained the Kabaka's aura of God-given invincibility.

One evening, I was called to the doctor's lounge. An armed

guard stood at the curtain of the lounge. He waved me in with the business end of whatever weapon he carried. I was surprised to see my consultant, Dr. Money, in the room. He was not on service, and in any case the consultant only came when called by the resident. I later learned that only a black physician could attend to this most important patient, the Katikiro of Buganda. Dr. Money, shortened from Monekoso, was Nigerian, not Ugandan, but no matter.

Dr. Money was bent over this heavy distressed man seated restlessly on an armchair that had been brought to this otherwise sparse room. His trousered legs were elevated on another chair, and his long white *kanzu* was opened at the neck.

Most alarmingly, the Katikiro's tongue was swollen several times its normal size and could no longer be contained in his mouth. Nurses mopped his predicament, both Dr. Money's and the Katikiro's. I stared. Dr. Money labeled it angioneurotic edema and expressed concern for his airway.

We pushed and shoved his chair with this impossibly heavy patient and his tongue into the only single room on the floor. His own effort got him onto the bed, and we kept his head elevated. Nightmares of his tongue falling back and forever and fatally obstructing his glottis passed through our minds.

The trouble was also his neck. None could be discerned. His head appeared to come straight out of his chest. A surgeon, this time Ugandan black, was called in case an intubation or a tracheostomy was required. I saw him searching anxiously for the Katikiro's neck. I could see his thoughts willing that no emergency occurred. In the days to come, I saw him several times in the room requesting the Katikiro to look upwards and stroking the tiny crevice between torso and head—searching, searching.

This was the land where witchcraft formed a strong alternative thread of reason and unreason. I heard whispers of how the enemies of the Katikiro via the *Shami*, the tribal medicine man, had zeroed their attack on the weapon the Katikiro used best—his tongue.

In spite of his discomfort, we dared not sedate him, lest drowsiness cause the catastrophe we feared. However, positive thoughts, epinephrine, antihistamines and possibly counter-*Shami* efforts worked, and his Excellency was soon conducting court from his hospital bed.

Roasted peanuts and a pool of tears

To mark the end of my internal medicine rotation, we took a trip to Fort Portal. Amir's mother and father, Ma and Bapa, wanted to participate in the celebration of the opening of the new Ismaili mosque We would combine this with a visit to Bapa's younger brother Badru, his wife Shirin, and Amir's paternal grandmother, who lived with Badru. My ulterior motive was to visit the Queen Elizabeth National Park around Lake George.

Amir drove and Bapa sat up in front, with Ma and me in the back seats. Ma constantly remarked on the peace and comfort of the present trip and compared it with the last time she had made this journey, though there was much discussion as to whether the last time her destination was Fort Portal or Mbarara. She specially emphasized how much she appreciated my slim body that took up so little space. On that other *safari*, she had sat in the back seat with her sister Shera *Masi* and friend Jenna *Masi*. The *Masi* after each name means 'Aunt,' indicating either a relationship or just a mark of respect. Jenna *Masi* was rail-thin, but Shera *Masi* had that plateau-like front that many older Ismaili women develop, different from their Parsi counterparts who develop those shelf-like bosoms on which to display diamond jewelry. Ma also had a comfortable figure with wide hips, convenient for the many babies she delivered without problem.

During this remembered journey, Shera *Masi*'s somewhat subdued and mild husband sat in the passenger seat with four-year-old Amir on his lap. Driving them was Seka Jugu, an African, whose name translated to Roasted Peanuts. From the start of the journey the ladies on the back seat grumbled and fretted over space. *'Jara agel beso'* — 'Please sit a little forward.' *'Jara sankra thao,'* literally, 'Please make yourself narrower.' This, though politely spoken, continued incessantly for several miles.

Finally Seka Jugu (Roasted Peanuts) could take it no more. He stopped the car in the wilderness, threw the car keys on the front seat and said he would rather walk home than tolerate a minute more of the quibbling women. Shera *Masi* was furious. The feast at the mosque they were visiting was to be made by her and she needed to get there on time. She demanded that her husband do something. Since the man did not drive, he was reduced to standing on the road and accosting the few passers-by, offering bribes to have the group driven. Finally a *matatu*—taxi—drove alongside. The driver refused to drive their car, but said he would get a friend to bring it later and was reluctantly given the key. A price for the ride was argued and bargained down till a fuming Shera *Masi* told her husband to stop being cheap. Her husband in turn said he would only enter the taxi and pay the fare if the three ladies kept total and complete silence for the rest of the trip. So in smoldering silence, using only body language to create their spaces, they reached their destination.

We reached Badru and Shirin's home and I met Dadi Ma—Amir's grandmother—for the first time. She had a cool presence, and her face spoke of an aquiline and long-ago beauty, crowned now with a silver bun. She greeted me gracefully, putting her hand on my head and giving a symbolic gift of a few shillings.

Later, in Gujerati, she described the making of the communal *biryani* on the grounds of the mosque. She appreciated and commented on how the men helped in the difficult task of cutting fifty pounds of onions, twenty pounds of potatoes and twenty pounds of goat's meat. Putting it together was easy, she said. It was the onion-cutting that was hard. In her day, she said, men would never help. To tarnish this enlightened perspective, she did emphasize that on occasions such as this, Africans should not be allowed to help or touch the food being prepared.

The next day, Amir drove them to the mosque in the morning for prayers and serious *biryani*-making. And then Amir and I took off for the game park named after Queen Elizabeth II. We drove a couple of hours south into the park and then took a spectacular boat ride through the Kazinga Channel connecting Lakes Edward and George.

The water near the shores of the lake was alive with feathers. A portend of the birds. And then the birds. Fearlessly standing on one or both legs, preening, staring, some expressing a sudden startling rattle. And they were large. Pelicans and storks. Herons of wide variety, green-backed, which I have since seen in my Ossining garden, black-headed and gray. Egrets and sacred ibis. And the carrion-eater hang-man maribou stork looking at you with a hard ironic unflinching gaze. Fish eagles perched on nearby trees gazing at the scene with you. And snake-necked cormorants and grebes. Flamingos tingeing all with sunset pink.

I did not have a camera, but what stayed with me is a likeness to the black-and-white Tenniel illustrations in Alice in Wonderland, the one where Alice having wept and wept caused a pool of tears to form. 'And the pool was getting quite crowded with the birds and animals that had fallen into it: there was a Duck and a Dodo, a Lory and an Eaglet, and several other curious creatures.' And innocent Alice leads the swimmers to the shore. But was she innocent? I recently saw photographs taken by Lewis Carroll of the original Alice Lidell. One in particular showed her sullen, sultry and sexy. I know I have not finished with understanding that book.

We completed our day at the restaurant of the hotel in Fort Portal and then had a second dinner of *biryani* at home while Ma and others regaled us with happenings at the gala dinner at the mosque.

Obstetrics and gynecology—Mulago style

On the last day of my Internal Medicine rotation we were making our usual professorial rounds. Slow, thoughtful and ... contemplative. We stopped at the bed of a young beautiful dark-eyed man whose right leg had been amputated. Professor Williams said he had received a letter from the patient's previous caregiver confirming that the leg had been amputated because of an embolus, a blood clot, which had originated from a damaged heart valve when the heart had maddened into a whirlwind arrhythmia. 'Who wrote the letter asking for the information?' he asked. I had. He turned his back to me and told the wall something that made me flush with pleasure. He said to the wall, 'What a shame Dr. Tejani is going to be wasted on Obstetrics.'

Why would he care? Decades later, I understand a trite quotation in Samson Wright's textbook of *Applied Physiology*. It went, 'More than the calf wants to suck does the cow yearn to suckle.' There are some students who listen with their hearts and they are unforgettable.

Well, too late to change course now. I had to plunge into Obstetrics and Gynecology. When and why did I make that decision? As blurred as the question people often ask—Why medicine? Nothing positive, no altruistic story of a sick or dying relative. Everything else just seemed too frivolous.

I had been warned that the Chairperson of Obstetrics and Gynecology was in the G mold. A daunting, missionary colonial variation on G. Professor Coralie Rendle-Short had spent her early years practicing Obstetrics in China. After her time in Uganda she was Professor and Chairperson in Addis Ababa, Ethiopia, and then in Korea. After retirement she studied religion and at the age of eighty-four was awarded a Ph.D. in theology. Clearly a remarkable woman. But I had to start from square one and do my best to make her rethink her *dukawalla* feelings about Asians. It took time but, to her credit, she eventually fostered and helped me along. Quite a long time.

Three of us entered into newly created positions specifically to train for the MRCOG degree in Obstetrics and Gynecology. There was Dr. F.M. Bulwa, portly, smiling, black, shining and a master surgeon, vastly experienced and capable of managing any surgical emergency. He told me that one night at a rural hospital in the *charo*, the tiny hospital where he worked lost electricity and he had to perform an emergency cesarean section. So the patient was carried on to the open verandah of the hospital and placed on the stone floor. He then swung his car around, shone the headlights on to the woman's belly and did the cesarean by car-light. He had someone adjust the lights by moving the car as needed. Fearless was he.

Then there was Gareth Barberton, tall and tanned and much at home with the rest of the colonial consultants, who trusted him completely. This could have been a 'one of us' thing, but it was also based on the extensive 'up country' experience he had before this assignment. On one occasion in the doctors' lounge adjoining the operating rooms, Professor Rendle-Short was being particularly shrill and oppressive with me. I had discovered a patient with a large ovarian tumor. It was her day to operate, and I could not contact her. Admittedly I did not try very hard because I found her a jumpy and nervous surgeon who did not mesh well with my inexperience. I did the case with Dr. Mary Tolley, a big gentle soft-spoken New Zealander. As the Professor raved, my eyes met Gareth's. And though no word was said, I realized his sympathy. And I thanked him, also without speaking.

So there we were—a black male, a white male and an Asian woman all working hard, often, literally, night and day, toward the same goal. What a wonderful and much-needed story of racial harmony we could have made together. But we did nothing toward that. During the day we were so busy that we seldom crossed paths. And come evening we parted ways—me to my blue haven and Asian family and friends, Gareth to his colonial hillside friends and Bulwa to the unseen *Charo*. I was not mature enough to see the opportunity for something much bigger than just doing the job.

No fetal heart

The story of the patient that I had caused the professor to miss was like this:
I had been called to the clinic as the midwives failed to find a fetal heart on this distressed teenager with an immensely pregnant silhouette. I palpated her abdomen and could not really get a grip on the fetus. Loss of amniotic fluid due to fetal demise, I said to

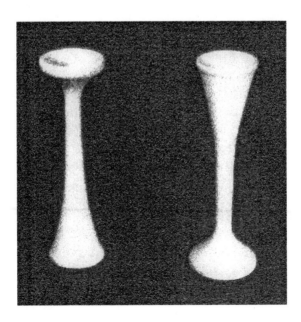

myself. No fetal heartbeat was heard through the trumpet-shaped device we used for the purpose. We sent the woman for an X-ray of the abdomen. A demise may be recognized on X-ray by a crumpled fetus assuming exaggerated postures it could never manage in life and overlapping of the skull bones as the brain dwindles in death. Strange gas shadows outline the fetal blood vessels as the contained blood surrenders its life-giving gases—a sign of no hope. A subtle diagnosis unlike today's real-time instantaneous recognition of absent heart motion on ultrasound.

But there was no fetus at all. Ugly shades of gray painted a large tumor. A tumor it was, but not a tumor of love. A more careful pelvic examination revealed a large ovarian mass pushing the small uterus aside.

'But,' exclaimed the puzzled patient, 'I have been coming to the clinic for two months!'

In embarrassment, I checked the records. Three visits were recorded, each one impossibly documenting a fetal heartbeat. Today, instrumentation loudly proclaims a heartbeat to all within earshot, including that most important witness, the mother. How to explain the fictitious heartbeat only heard by the examiner? How to explain that in medical nights there are teeming deceptions, most passing unnoticed, some harmful, most harmless, but deceptions nevertheless. Hearts of darkness everywhere. Reading Conrad's Kurtz brought me pangs of recognition. So many unconfirmable events to twist and turn, blurring the truth. A heart of darkness in all of us, specially that tired overextended medico.

I stammered some explanation. She needed surgical exploration and removal of the mass. I made a date with her.

'I have told everyone that I am pregnant,' she says. 'Never will I go back and tell this new tale. I'm staying in the hospital till it is done. Then', she adds, 'I'll go home and tell them I have had a stillbirth.' Sadly, with fetal and newborn mortality several hundred-fold that in the developed world, this would be a reasonable and believable story. Better a stillbirth that all would sympathize with, rather than this ridiculous ovarian tumor. So I booked the case for the next morning. That's when I half-heartedly searched for the Professor and happily called Dr.Tolley when I failed to find her.

She was anesthetized and opened via a maximal mid-line

incision from xiphi-sternum to pubic bones. A giant ovarian tumor had taken over the right ovary. The rest of her abdomen looked clean and free. No ugly evidences of a cancer that had spread. Peritoneal fluid sent for emergent testing showed no cancer cells. A simple excision of the ovary and tube followed. Too easy. She would never know the difference.

The cut surface of the tumor showed multiple cystic and solid areas, many darkened with old blood. Days later a pathology report confirmed a granulosa cell tumor, a slow-growing minimally malignant tumor involving the ovarian follicles that nurse future eggs.

For further and more specific identification, the clear spaces—Call-Exner bodies—were reported as present. That nostalgic old medical practice of calling things by the names of the person(s) who first described them. Call and Exner poring over primitive microscopes, together? Independently? Racing for publication to be the first with immortal names. Males? Females? Strangers? Friends? In love? Mr. Call and Ms. Exner.

On the third day after surgery, the patient called out to me and said, 'Look at this.' She squeezed her breast and out poured an arc rivaling the Milky Way.

'This can only happen after a baby,' she stated with 'I told you so' in her eyes. A granulosa cell tumor involves cells that secrete estrogen and progesterone. I started trying to explain, but stopped.

I included this case in the book we had to prepare for our board examinations. In it I hypothesized several convoluted reasons for lactation after removal of a granulosa cell tumor. Estrogen, progesterone, prolactin.

Perhaps it was nothing more mysterious than an anguished heart wishing for a believable story when she got back. I offered to help suppress lactation with medication. She refused adamantly and left hastily, sooner than anticipated, to reach home with her evidence intact.

The Bantu pelvis

Our professor Coralie gave her three trainees weekly tutorials. In one, she reinforced standard teaching on the classic pelvic types and then told us that this did not apply here in Uganda.

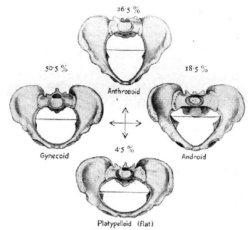

CHARACTER INLET OF THE FOUR PARENT TYPES OF PELVIS.
(Caldwell and Moloy.)

We memorized the old stodgy types of pelves—gynecoid, android, anthropoid and platypelloid. But no one had written about this little frill—a frill of a pelvis.

Just as in India we had learnt about all the glorified and corrupt Henrys and Jameses and Wars of Independence that were twisted into Indian mutinies—and just as in Africa we learnt of the beneficence of Christianity and the value of multiple Victorian petticoats to cover bare bodies in Equatorial climates—so we learnt of the inapplicable pelvis.

First, that perfectly shaped gynecoid pelvis. A perfect Valentine heart at the brim and a generous arch under the pubic bones, ischial spines on the sides that were so flush they could not even be felt. A smooth ride for the little one or even a big one. Then the android pelvis that was designed for a forever-barren male. A sharp triangle instead of a sweetheart for the brim, with its most generous diameter so far back that it was unusable for the little passenger. With its side walls coned inwards and with a narrow pubic arch and threatening ischial spines, it was a veritable maze for the innocent. Even a death trap if left too long. Third was the anthropoid pelvis with its emphasis on the front-back diameters with miserable side-to-sides. A fetus in its endorphic state is supposed to know to negotiate this peril facing either directly forward or directly backward. The last prototype was the platypelloid pelvis, which is the anthropoid rotated so that the widest measurements are from side to side. The fetal head comes down in this generous transverse diameter. Low and exposed before your eyes, it makes that forward rotation that is usually secret and unseen. Platypelloid reveals all.

But what was this frill of a pelvis? A band, no more. So shallow that the fetal head could be visualized even when it had not even entered the brim—not even started its pelvic journey. We tried the North American introduction of expressing the descent of the fetal head in stations, but these terms groped without meaning. The landmark 'zero' station did not mean that the widest diameter of the fetal head had engaged the brim of the pelvis—far from it. At 'zero' station it had often not even started the pelvic journey.

And there was yet another wonder. The direction of the pelvic canal in the standing position was directly backwards—parallel to the horizontal. The baby had to swing around this bend to reach us. There were advantages to this arrangement. The traditional *dingi-dingi* dance, where the hips swing fast and wild, was much facilitated and effortless, thanks to this natural tilt and lilt. Prolapse and relaxation of the pelvic organs was a rarity because backward angulation of the pelvis caused the weight of the abdominal organs to fall against the abdominal wall rather than the vaginal, urethral or rectal openings. All those protracted labors, sometimes for days, but no genital prolapse.

Having always been myopic, the crystal moments I remember are of smell and sounds and touch. I remember the smell of sweet-peas in a long-forgotten garden that my mother tended. Each year I try to bring them back, but I never equal those sweet nodding fragrances of memory. I remember the first touch of a wet and slippery newborn against my inner thigh—three events rolled into one, at that exhilarating end of the second stage of labor.

And I will forever remember that crack. The crack of the pubic bones separating, tough cartilage tearing.

She was a teenager, pregnant for the first time, who was admitted in labor. She had read the book on cervical dilatation and followed Eli Friedman's cervical dilatation rules dutifully—till she was fully dilated and the fetal head stopped cold at the ischial spines. The usual chorus of 'Sindika, sindika'—'Push, push'—produced no results. A cesarean section, I thought. The consultant had a golf date, but came in. Dr. Derek Scotland had white hair that belied a youthful face, effacing, quiet, with a permanent bland smile. He had done what he was about to do many times before.

'Let's help her permanently, enlarge her pelvis forever,' he said.

Her legs were raised to the 'obstetric' position and local nerve blocks given. Slim Kielland's forceps were slid onto the fetal head, which lay transversely in this little pelvis. It was a perfect cephalic application, but there was no way to rotate and extract it without causing injury.

'Support the forceps blades in place,' I was instructed. More local anesthetic was injected above and behind the pubic bones and a centimeter-long incision was made above the pubic bones. A space was created behind the pubic bones and a solid scalpel—I have not seen one in decades—was inserted into the created space. The cartilage between the pubic bones was located and patiently sawed through. As the end approached, a person on each side held her hips together and then slowly let them fall apart. Then that CRACK, forever held in some part of my memory.

It worked! The pelvic bones separated and rotated outwards unhampered by the pubic symphysis joint that had held them together. At least 2cms was gained in the transverse diameter of the pelvis. Smooth and easy traction and rotation low on the pelvic floor resulted in a fine baby.

'Do we have to put the joint back together?'

'No', said Dr. Scotland, 'The pubic symphysis carries no weight. Weight passes from the vertebral column outwards along the pelvic bones to and through the hip joints into the legs.' Unbelievable! And probably untrue.

I tried to explain this to the patient when she would not or could not walk the next day. I told her of the permanent benefit to her pelvis. She remained unimpressed.

Over the course of a week she did get up and walk, a strange rolling walk. And then she walked right out of our lives.

Did she live to dance and deliver again? Neither my golfing consultant nor I would ever know.

1961: GC Day

Determined to make us as academic as possible, Coralie gave us one study day a week. Often, as a result of sleep deprivation, I would just sleep that Thursday away. Other days I would take my books and spend the day in Amir's 'surgery,' eavesdropping on what went on.

Streams of patients would come in with the complaint 'I have a cold in my urethra'—the euphemism for gonorrhea—commonly shortened to GC (for gonococcus). How do you know? 'Pus, pain. I got it from my wife who got it from her first man. I have given it to my girlfriend.' Nobody stopped to confirm the diagnosis. Any one of the town's docs would give the patient penicillin. One shot, or two if he could afford it, to cover possible syphilis. Sulphadiazine if he could only produce pennies or a pineapple. At the time, the gonococcus responded to even a whiff of penicillin.

When I needed to take a break, I would walk around the crowded neighborhood. On the corner where the taxi stop merged in confusion with the bus stop I saw a local 'doctor' displaying his wares. On a tarp set on the dust there were bottles containing twigs and leaves. In others, some distinctly animal-looking products— furry skin scraps and claws. What did they cure? The medicine man slept sitting upright near his merchandise, unavailable for consultation. Sunlight glinted on a glass container in the corner of his display. It was a grubby penicillin vial half filled with grayish fluid, expiration date long passed. A salute to Alexander Fleming, maybe even the original mold.

It was not just a cold. Repeated infections caused painful urethral strictures in the male, obstructing the passage of urine, eventually causing back pressure and permanent kidney damage. In women, acute pelvic infections forever disorganized the order of the pelvis. Fallopian tubes closed to the passage of ova. Tubes distorted and entrapped embryos instead of allowing safe passage to the cushiony uterus, causing life-threatening tubal pregnancies. Tubes swollen into pus-filled receptacles threatening to rupture—a potentially fatal situation. And tubes converted into dilated retort-shaped uselessness. All the perverse ways of the gonococcus— smooth bean-shaped couplets of bacteria—staining bright red and devastating the pelvis.

A specialist arrived from Iceland. The title of his talk was 'How gonorrhea was abolished in Iceland,' making the speaker redundant.

He started with the preliminaries. The history of the organism and infection, clinical presentations, pathologic diagnosis. And then the management. Circumstances peculiar to Iceland included a sparse population, limited travel in and out of the country, and, as in Uganda, complicated and innumerable contacts.

His solution was unique. He had talked the government into proclaiming a national holiday—GC day. On that day, everyone, but everyone, was to receive a shot of penicillin. It had to be timed narrowly so that 'contact' between treated and untreated was unlikely. Like Armistice Day observed on 11/11 at 11 minutes past 11 a.m. Everyone saddens at the same time, remembering our war dead.

A question and answer period followed.

'Penicillin allergies?' 'Discount—just inject.'

'Serious reactions?' 'None.'

'Syphilis would be incompletely treated by this regime.' 'Eradicating syphilis was not the goal.'

'Who gave the shots?' 'Staff went to each settlement and trained volunteers who ended the session by injecting each other.'

'Who financed?' 'Government, from assessments of gambling establishments'—at least I think that is what he said. I never heard of casinos in Iceland, so I may have misheard.

It appeared that the cost was drop-dead reactions and progressing masked syphilis.

A discussion ensued, and it was resolved to hold yet another discussion. Another meeting was held with dwindling attendance. This required organization and determination, volunteers and funding. Dangerous allergic reactions and syphilis became the euphemisms for inaction.

For some years Uganda has become a model amongst African countries for reducing HIV rates without expensive medication. Uganda's President Museveni was welcomed to the White House and asked to share the secret of his success. 'The ABC method,' he said. 'Abstinence. Be faithful. And Condoms.' George Bush loved the A and the B. But I do believe it was the C that did it.

Tubo-ovarian abscess

The gonococcus (GC) is a wily enemy. In the female its initial inception and infection is subtle but, unlike the male, it is not painful. Anything that is not painful can slide in unnoticed. It obtains access quietly, sexually, through an infected male partner. And its first serious stop is the cervix, the mouth of the uterus. A lesser stop may be the gland whose secretion lubricates the vagina—Bartholin's gland—which is announced by pain and inflammation and often an abscess. It can lie unseen amongst all the luxuriant folds and crevices of the cervix, sometimes totally silent but often manifesting as a purulent discharge. As yet it has not reached places where it can really cause havoc, and this is an optimal time for intervention.

Presently, it is standard care to screen all pregnant women for GC when they first seek prenatal care. It is a peculiar but happy fact that the GC usually (but not always) goes no further in pregnancy and has the decency to delay its journey at the cervix—rest a while. The problem in pregnancy is that during vaginal delivery, intimate contact with the fetus may infect its eyes. If not appropriately treated, this can be serious. I once read that the main cause of blindness in children in the middle ages was GC infection of the eyes—ophthalmitis—following vaginal delivery through an infected cervix.

The GC is reticent during pregnancy, but outside pregnancy it is ruthless. It travels up into the uterus, but, probably because the lining of the uterus is shed on a monthly basis, it does not waste its energies here. It finds the pinhole openings of the Fallopian tubes into the uterus, one at each cornu of the uterus, and then it has a field day of uncontrolled excesses. It infects the tubes, first without scarring and still reversible with antibiotics. If not checked, it causes scarring and tubal blockage usually at its distal end, causing it to swell into an abscess. It may do other nasty things as well, but the tubo-ovarian abscess is its greatest treachery. A bad guest's attempt to kill its host...or hostess.

Our gynecologic ward was a large hall crammed with patients on basic steel beds and on the floor between beds. The main reasons for hospital admission were manifold variations on the infected pelvis, some complication of the all-pervasive fibroid uterus, vesico-vaginal fistula and cancers, most commonly advanced cancer of the cervix. But pelvic infections predominated. The trick was to treat conservatively with antibiotics, but have an acute awareness if a tubo-ovarian abscess had formed. This would not respond unless treated surgically—like any abscess, the pus needs to be let out and drained. Optimal treatment is what we arrogantly call a clean-out—removal of the damaged uterus, tubes and ovaries. But we had to blend practice with the wishes of the patients we treated. Not to menstruate in an Ugandan woman of reproductive age was unacceptable to her, and we endeavored never to remove the damaged organs.

This is the summary of a record from my MRCOG 'book' of a case of ruptured tubo-ovarian abscess and presently outdated surgical management. But the patient survived.

On the 23rd of July 1961, Mariam N, a 33-year-old Muganda woman, was admitted to Mulago Hospital for high fevers, severe lower abdominal pain, pain with passing urine and a purulent vaginal discharge. She had also noticed a mass in the lower abdomen which was now tender and painful.

The patient stated that she had been experiencing pain over a gradually increasing lower abdominal mass for six years but that it had intensified over the last 24 hours. She had never sought any help for this. Also, over the last eleven days, she had high intermittent fevers.

She had one child eleven years of age and was concerned about never conceiving again.

When admitted, her vital signs were stable and she had a temperature of 102 degrees. There was discharge from the cervix which tested positive for GC. Tender masses were palpated in the lower abdomen, the left being the larger and the right the size of 'an orange.' So much easier and more objective to use approximated dimensions but the inexplicable habit of using fruit for descriptive terms persists till today.

A diagnosis of tubo-ovarian abscesses was made and the patient was admitted, hydrated and placed on the antibiotics of the day— penicillin and streptomycin.

At 6.15 that evening, a dramatic change occurred in her condition. Her pain had increased and she appeared ill and toxic.

Her blood pressure had dropped, and her heart rate was up to 140 beats per minute. There were generalized signs of peritonitis, and her abdomen was very tender, responding to any touch by 'guarding,' a protective contraction of the abdominal muscles because of pain. We correctly guessed that the worst complication of tubo-ovarian abscess had occurred, that it had ruptured. This condition carried a mortality of over 50 percent. Surgery was now her only chance at survival.

An hour later, she was in the operating room under general anesthesia. A large vertical abdominal incision confirmed the worst. A 'melon-sized' left tubo-ovarian abscess and an 'orange-sized' right one. Both had ruptured and three 'pints' of foul-smelling pus had flooded the abdomen. It is a strange fact in this business that when I am literally steeped in this fetid material, as long as it is in the right place—an operating room—I have absolutely no reaction to it. I would swoon if I smelt this in my kitchen, which makes me guess that everything is 'right' in its own place. All this purulent material was suctioned off and the abdomen washed with copious amounts of saline. Part of the necrotic left (the melon) was removed and the tube tied off at its uterine end. The pus from the right tube (the orange) was also drained and the tube tied at its uterine end.

The tying off of tubes at their uterine end was called the Falk procedure after an American gynecologist. His thesis was that causing a discontinuity between the uterus and the tube would discourage the infection, usually gonorrheal as it was in my patient, from traveling up the uterus from the cervix to re-infect the tubes. This seemed like an excellent solution for our patients as it involved minimal and relatively simple surgery as compared to a formidable hysterectomy in the face of distortions and adhesions. Additionally it kept intact the menstrual function of the uterus which was so important to the patient. Years later in the U.S., I discovered that this surgical procedure had been long discarded as the retained organs were a constant source of re-infection and cure was not effected till the damaged tissue and uterus were removed.

It is dismaying to think upon the numerous false beliefs we have practiced innocently and erroneously. Most were harmless and some harmful. Many examples come to mind. At one time we were convinced that, in the newborn, oxygen was absorbed as easily from the stomach lining as it was from the lungs. This required the passage of a tube into the stomach to deliver the oxygen, a simple matter, rather than the much more complicated tube into the trachea. We practiced this for some time before it dawned on us that the premise was incorrect and the newborn in need of oxygen could absorb it from no other site than its lungs. Many babies were lost or damaged as a result of this misconception. Less harmful was the teaching that all preterm babies should be delivered with obstetric forceps. The theory was that a protective iron cage around the head would protect the soft and vulnerable head from injury. If properly applied this method of delivery at least caused no harm. And some good came of it since the trainees became exquisitely skillful at the procedure—presently another art lost at the altar of that all-pervasive cesarean section.

Back to the patient. Rubber drainage tubes were placed on either side and the abdomen was closed. It speaks to the fortitude of our patient that she made a remarkable recovery, was taking oral nourishment by the fourth postoperative day and was recovered sufficiently a week later to be sent home.

I made no note of any follow-up. I presume almost certainly that it would recur and that someday, unknown to me, she would return even more sick. Even the obvious—tracking down her contact and treating him for gonorrhea—was beyond the scope of our practice, which was too busy to do anything other than attend to problems that had already occurred as best we could, and give no thought to prevention.

Gifting a disease

An old story is told of Babur, the first of the great Mughal emperors, sitting by the bedside of his ailing son Humayun in the waning days of his rule. After some contemplation he walked around the sick bed three times, willing his son's ailment to enter into him--a death wish that, because of his power, was realized. Babur died and Humayun ruled for many glorious years.

Not all disease-gifting myths are altruistic. Gonorrhea and its sequelae were widespread in the young male Ugandan population, and there was a pernicious myth that intercourse with a virgin girl would rid the man of his disease. Successfully infecting the girl was thought essential to the cure, as the victim was often brought in by the rapist who was anxious to know if she had gonorrhea. As feeling grew against this practice I saw fewer of the openly exultant rapists.

One afternoon I was called to the Emergency Room for a 'rape case.' As I entered the barracks-like ER, I noticed two children, a girl and a boy, playing together on the grassy slope outside. I asked for the patient, and a woman in traditional dress called out to the child outside who was her daughter. She toddled in—all of three years of age. This was going to be particularly hard. Three years old and already caught in this malevolence.

After delaying the inevitable with history taking and questions, with the mother's help I positioned the child for examination. The child lay uncomplainingly in the dorsal lithotomy position—on her back with legs apart and raised. So composed was she that I could not help but think that she had done this before. She was relaxed and quiet and alarmingly easy to examine. Almost at once I saw a small clean-looking laceration from her vaginal opening back toward her rectum. A clean almost surgical incision, like the midline episiotomy I had made so many times to facilitate delivery.

Her quiet demeanor continued through the examination that involved insertion of a child-sized speculum, the taking of specimens for sperm and evidence of infection and digital pelvic examination with one finger. I called the mother to my end of the examining table to show her the laceration which would require repair. She said she had seen it and wanted me to go ahead with the repair. I noticed she spoke perfect English whereas till now she had communicated with me in Luganda through an interpreter. She quietly informed me that she was a nurse in a local mission hospital.

After preparing the child I sutured the little laceration in three layers using a local numbing agent. Once again she flinched not. I rapidly completed the surgery with absorbable sutures so that she would not need to have them removed. In those days, before the availability of synthetic sutures, we used plain catgut, an animal product that caused some swelling and inflammation but usually dissolved within a week and fell out leaving healing tissue.

At the end of the repair she got up, allowed her mother to dress her and went back to her playmate on the grassy verge.

I asked the mother if she knew who could be the perpetrator of this. Her black sad eyes settled on me for a few moments. She then vaguely pointed in the direction of the girl's playmate. Also a three-year-old.

'Cousin,' she whispered, her eyes still engaging mine. I half got up from my chair to go toward the little boy and then prevented myself from this absurdity.

A secret she could not tell lay behind this. The reason why the child appeared entirely acclimatized to being touched and probed. A reason for the mother's sad eyes that cried without shedding a tear. A reason that the woman had to protect beyond all consideration of safety for her child. A reason beyond all decency.

Version clinic

My days varied from labor room coverage, gynecologic surgery, Coralie's tutorials. But whatever it was, if we had time, we went down to the prenatal clinics.

These clinics were loud, funny and incessant. A picnic atmosphere prevailed. They started when the patients arrived and ran all day every weekday. Several comfortable-bodied nursing aides ran the encounter rooms. Nurses, midwives and any Ob/Gyn doctors who were not occupied elsewhere saw patients assembly-line style in a large hall with curtained cubicles. The crowds never abated and after the examination, patients often lounged on the grass outside under the shade of a friendly mango tree with their homemade *matoke* and sauce, to hear about each other's pregnancies.

The scene outside the clinic was often photographed. Shiny-faced women dressed in *basutis* of every hue were alive with a pregnancy glow. The *basuti* is an unlikely costume for tropical Africa. Long and wrapped, brightly hued cotton, often with words of advice or pure fun written over them. 'Hide your man from young women,' 'Don't go with a man without teeth.' 'Dancing is better than crying.' Although tightly wrapped, the effect was far from sleek because of the layers of striped petticoats—which served as bedding when needed—leg-o-mutton sleeves and an obi-styled sash holding it all together. Victoriana, Baganda style. It was difficult to match these beauties with the morbidity and mortality in the labor and delivery unit. But they were probably a different group of women. It was the old story of prenatal care being lavished on those who do not need it, while the needy, problem-ridden woman lurked alone in the shadows.

At the prenatal clinic, lining up at the blue door, were women waiting for versions—turning the fetus. Their fetuses, on palpation, were presenting buttocks first, a breech presentation. Our instructions were to turn them to a head presentation at any gestational age after 32 weeks. This may occur spontaneously, but since the patients may not return for care, and often deliver at home attended by traditional birth attendants, a fetal head presenting was safer. I was amused to see, in a 2003 paper in the *Green* journal, an article advocating versions at early gestational ages as though it wasa new concept--as we had practiced so many decades ago.

When I first came to New York in the early 70's, I discovered that version was regarded as a dangerous practice and breech presentation was an indication for cesarean section. The origin of this thinking was a paper describing several serious complications associated with version. Silent nostalgia brought back to me the hundreds that were performed by us without incident on those sunny clinic days. Better not to rock the boat when I was on that treacherous North American learning curve. Somebody later told me that the writer of the paper describing dire outcomes from versions had the physique of a football player and had to succeed no matter what. Gentle, gentle, I remember my teachers telling me, and know when to give up. Version is presently 'in' in the U.S., and everyone has become an expert after years of never using it.

Version clinics were my favorite. First stop, bathroom, to empty the bladder. Lay the woman down and get a good feel for the fetus—no sonogram to extend your hands. As I look back there must have been head presentations mistaken for breech that were turned into breech presentations. I heard that there was a notorious gentleman called Potter from Buffalo, NY, who routinely did this. The rationale could only be guessed at.

Anyway, get a good feel for the fetus. Confirm the round head above and the structureless soft buttocks presenting. Determine the side of the continuous smooth firm fetal back. Confirm a fetal heartbeat. Rotate the fetus into a forward somersault. maintaining flexion—bending—always maintaining flexion. Never unfold the primal fetal position. The initial dislodging is always a little difficult, but once eased, held and encouraged slowly in the right direction, the rest often just whizzed into a head-first position.

Prop the patient's head up for a few minutes to stabilize the fetal head. Fetal heart OK—next, please.

Anemia, African style

Coralie and the books taught us that anemia in the pregnant woman was most commonly due to iron deficiency because of the increased iron requirements of the mother and fetus. Next in line was a large-celled anemia caused by folic acid deficiency. And then a host of rarer anemias due to an inherent fragility of the red blood cells. But this was Africa, and we had to reword all these dogmas.

Her skin was a color without a name. Overtly black but now without shine or smile. Stone dull gray is closest. The inside of her mouth was dirty white. Her conjunctivae were the color of my doctor's coat. Her palms were plaster white. Also thirty-seven weeks pregnant.

'I'm tired,' she said.

This was no ordinary anemia. 'Let's test your blood.' No problem with the phlebotomy. But I looked up at her when I see what is collecting in the syringe. Watery pink-colored—no semblance to the real thing. A manual measurement in an old-styled Hemoglobinometer showed a value of three grams—barely measurable. Just a touch of red in a sea of fluid.

How was she sustaining herself? More miraculous, how was she providing for her little parasite fetus? I examine her belly. The fetus was the expected size with a reassuring heartbeat.

This is a symbiotic relationship, till there are problems. Then the little one has to adapt and live by its wits to cope with its hostile and unrelenting oxygen-poor atmosphere. It does many desperate things.

It pours out erythropoetin—a hormone—in response to the depleted oxygen that its mother can barely afford to part with, to expedite the manufacture of new red blood cells. This top-speed production occurs mainly in the fetal bone marrow, but other sites are also recruited. The liver, the spleen, the placenta are all enrolled and enlarged with new vessels and blood-forming activity. The fetus steps up its speed of circulation. An excellent system of increased fetal oxygen affinity pre-exists and is accentuated in adversity. Under duress, the fetus snaps up any oxygen it sees at the placental exchange site. A reversion to the Paleolithic slime where tadpoles happily extracted traces of oxygen from murky water because of their phenomenal affinity for it.

In our setting, infestation with hookworm caused these severest anemias. These parasites gain entry through unshod feet and after a circuitous bodily route, eventually lodge in the intestines where they feast on the host's blood, resulting in these impressive anemias. The toxic medications needed for these parasites travel unimpeded to the fetus and therefore cannot be used in pregnancy. As a side effect, they also cause an initial lowering of the blood count, which these severely anemic patients cannot afford or tolerate.

A blood transfusion was needed, but extra volume would further strain her heart into failure.

Therefore, a laborious exchange transfusion, where her watery blood would be discarded and replaced in small quantities by red-cell-rich donor blood. With no mechanization this was done at the bedside with a large syringe and wide bore needle. Blood was run in through one secure vein, and as it ran in, her blood was withdrawn and discarded in equal amounts from another vein. This was a messy sticky bloody business that took hours. It had to be slow so as not to overload the heart, but faster than the blood-sucking hookworms. We continued till her hemoglobin was a luxurious 6 grams (normal 14 grams).

Toward the end of the transfusion she grimaced and announced that she was in labor. A rapid progression to full dilatation followed. An easy slither of a birth with minimal bleeding resulted in a lusty healthy parasite demanding to be fed.

A newborn hemoglobin of—shame on you—12 grams!

A gyn case

Kampala was the capital city, but really a small town. It had one main road with several side streets lined with small mainly Indian-owned stores. The owners of these businesses were the much-reviled *dukawallas* of G and Coralie. But their work habits, if not work ethics, were impeccable. Stores opened at the crack of dawn and closed after dark. But they always closed for an hour at lunchtime, and therein lies my story.

The Indian owner of a fabric store closed for lunch as usual at 12 noon. Unknown to him, his young Indian salesman and a Mugandan woman clerk did not leave. The two had taken special notice of each other in the days previously and had decided on this lunch-hour tryst with looks and a few words. They did not have much time for decorum since the owner would be back soon. They proceeded to make love under one of the counters.

The owner unlocked the door an hour later and was greeted by this unusual sight under the 'remnants for sale' counter. His two employees were locked in an oblivious embrace. At first he turned his wrath on the young Indian man invoking shame, religion, etc. The young man helplessly turned his head to the owner and said he could not escape. The woman appeared to be in a trance with legs and arms clamped around him, eyes closed and mouth clenched. Tentative attempts to release her vice-like grip only caused her to tighten further. Vaginismus! An old diagnosis that seems to have lost popularity.

Mr. P, the owner, thought he needed help. He walked over to the next store to request consultation. Mr. P, the *panwalla*, obliged, and the two Ps surveyed the situation. After some thought, they called the Fire Department. The Fire Department was called in for many unusual situations other than fires. Snakes were a common reason. But this!

The fire truck arrived. The large bluff British fire chief stomped in wearing a pair of size 18 boots, and made the decision to 'load it as is' onto a stretcher and take it to Mulago Hospital for resolution. His assistants loaded the problem — all eight limbs and two heads — onto a stretcher, strapped it in, threw a blanket over it and moved off, siren blaring, to the emergency department of Mulago Hospital.

The Emergency Room doctor considered the problem and after some thought decided it was a gynecologic case. In the days before the page system I received a written message delivered by a leering messenger which said, '2.45 p.m.—Sexual problem—Gyn consultation requested.' Another rape, I thought, though the message was unusually worded.

I walked over to the Emergency Room. It was a long ward with curtains separating patients' beds. I felt a snickering hushed atmosphere. I parted the curtains and entered the cubicle that was pointed out.

Confusion—two heads, one surely male—and then the full impact. The man, now in tears, locked in the vice-like limbs. The woman trembling, sweating but oblivious to words, to entreaties, to threats. I was young and sexually somewhat naive. This was not in my repertoire. This was surely a consultant's case.

I left the patient(s) to call my consultant. A small crowd gathered around me as I tried to explain the historical facts and specially the physical findings. The consultant, who was often difficult to get, came in without any trouble. He walked around the patients and tried gingerly, unsuccessfully, to pry them apart.

He had a bright idea and we called an anesthetist. A male nurse anesthetist walked in almost immediately—he must have been one of the spectating crowd. He displayed no emotion. We were all behaving as though we knew what we were doing. He prepared to intubate if necessary while I injected the sodium pentothal.

Gradually she relaxed. Fell apart. Somehow, at this moment, this somewhat comic situation ceased to be funny. The poor man, released, crept away. What will he feel if he and I ever meet again in this small small town? How will he live in this close-knit, exclusive, gossip-ridden Asian community?

The woman fell into a deep sleep. In the days that followed, she was treated for exhaustion, dehydration and a temporary renal shutdown—similar to the aftermath of widespread muscle injury. She recovered and left.

I heard later that she had set up 'shop' in Wandegaya, a mostly African-owned business area in the valley between Mulago and the Makerere hills. Only the most adventure-hungry males took her on.

The book

The book. The book. In hushed and reverent terms, we were introduced to what was an initiation rite equal to a Masai warrior entering manhood by killing a lion with only a spear, the first step toward our qualification. At different times in the last four decades I have picked up this 379-page tome bound in midnight blue and lettered in gold.

Gold letters on the cover say:

CASE RECORDS AND COMMENTARIES
BY NERGESH A. TEJANI

The 'A' was for Amir and well did he deserve mention in the book. We, he and I, paid to have it typed with red headers and black print—not an easy proposition when you remember that messy ink-soaked ribbons had to be changed to accomplish this. All the typographic errors were carefully corrected in his fine small script, much neater than my illegible scrawl.

On moving to Ossining, New York, in 1990, I found it in a box of books and left it out amongst other books on the coffee table. I was often surprised to see visitors of all ages and persuasions raptly absorbed in it. When I have looked at the pages over the years, I have had different reactions. Sometimes I am acutely embarrassed at the antiquated language, the qualitative terms, the lack of science and objectivity. At other times I am struck by how little has changed. And yet other times I have recognized that the cases are a truthful and unembellished commentary on life—and death—of the indigent in East Africa. This must be the reason for people paying such attention to it.

One of the astonishing descriptions was the obstetric pelvic examination. Each examination was preceded by a long, almost apologetic explanation for why the examination was performed, often planned in advance and then reluctantly performed. I quote '... the patient was asked to void urine as a vaginal exam was planned. After scrubbing with soap and water for five minutes and donning a sterile mask, gown and dry gloves, the vulvae were swabbed out with Hibitane in Cetrimide solution, the swabbing being carried out from before backwards toward the anus, each swab being used only once. A sterile towel was then placed under the patient. The labia majora having been cleaned, they were separated with the fingers of the left hand, and the vaginal opening was swabbed down in a similar manner. A substantial quantity of Dettol cream was taken on the fingers of the right hand and the index and middle fingers were inserted into the vagina.' Phew!

And today it is straight from McDonald's to the pelvic exam.

But then, our fingers felt things that we no longer care for. At the end of the preparatory ritual, listen to the description of the pelvic examination.

'The introitus was lax and elastic. The vagina was normal. The cervix was two and a half fingers (5 cms) dilated and well taken up (effaced). Membranes were present, and the presenting vertex was in the right occipito-transverse position, the anterior parietal bone presenting, slightly deflexed but well applied to the cervix. It was stationed just above the pelvic brim. No cord was felt.

'The sacral promontory was just reached (the true conjugate was estimated to be 9.8 cms). The sacrum was short and had a gentle curve. The inlet felt of the normal gynecoid type. The sacro-sciatic notches admitted two fingers. The ischial spines were not prominent. The rest of the mid-cavity felt normal. Retro-pubic and sub-pubic angles were adequate as were the transverse and posterior sagittal diameters of the outlet. On the whole, therefore, the pelvis was a well-rounded Bantu type. Cephalo-pelvic disproportion was tested for, and the (fetal) head could be pushed into the pelvic brim easily.' A forgotten art. Perhaps best forgotten.

We had to submit twenty obstetric and twenty gynecologic cases, each with a short commentary. And there they were. The eclamptics, the ruptured uteri, the huge perinatal mortality, the destructive fetal surgeries to avoid cesarean section in already dead babies, the deaths, deaths, deaths.

And the ectopics—at least one a day—tubo-ovarian abscesses of every size and shape, about to rupture and ruptured, fibroids in every nook and corner, exotic sexually transmitted diseases—*lympho-granuloma venereum*—and obstetric injury causing vesico-vaginal fistulae, an opening between the urinary bladder and the vagina, causing constant incontinence of urine.

My obstetric commentary was on the transverse lie in labor. Suffice it to say that of the 44 cases described, 6 mothers died of infection, hemorrhage, or ruptured uterus. There was a perinatal loss of 31 of 44, with many patients admitted neglected and infected with a fetal demise. The delivery methods were internal version and breech extraction, classical and lower-segment cesarean sections, and 11 babies, already dead, delivered by decapitation and extraction. Many moons and suns ago.

My gynaecologic commentary was a description of 'post-operative complications following 844 cases of abdominal gynaecological surgery with a mortality of 9 (i.e., 1%) from peritonitis, hemorrhage, anesthesia, and—most ominous of all—'unknown.' My analysis led to the conclusion that of the 9 deaths, 2 were unavoidable, 2 possibly avoidable, and 5 avoidable. A certain frankness and openness about this confession has to appreciated. Fear of litigation had not yet reared its querulous head.

The first page is stamped 'Accepted for MRCOG examination.' Retrospective, observational, uncontrolled as it was, I realized how much I enjoyed investigational work.

Eclampsia

I looked down at my right index finger in disbelief. It was a reflexive action without the intervention of common sense. I saw the seizure coming and had been taught to insert something, anything, between the patient's teeth to prevent injury to her tongue. But my right index finger? A right index finger is golden to an obstetrician. The pelvic examination is a staple. The right index and middle fingers are our main diagnostic tools. To feed it into a clamped jaw is beyond belief. Once between the teeth, a ray of good sense told me to keep it there till the end of the seizure and not to drag it out, which may have caused a shuddering injury. It was the longest seizure I have ever witnessed, and I certainly watched it from an intimate distance. No sympathy from my colleagues as they had to take on extra work because of my rashness. The blued nail and deep tooth-marked skin looked pitiful, but a tetanus shot later, healed.

I had been assigned to the eclampsia ward. Our Professor taught that preeclampsia did not occur in these Bantu lands, but eclampsia did. I think that we just did not recognize the beast till the seizure occurred.

The eclampsia unit consisted of a row of hospital beds in a darkened room. A toxic cocktail—demarol, phenargen and thorazine—ran intravenously in all patients in an unregulated flow—X drops per minute were the orders. The quiet sedated women had tongue depressors and airways at their sides. This was a disease of first pregnancies so the women in the row were young. The Swahili yarn was to get it over with in a first pregnancy and it will never happen again. The first time is like an immunization making you invulnerable for life.

The patient in 'three' had convulsed repeatedly before being conveyed to the hospital. Semi-conscious on arrival, she was further sedated to the point of apnea with our unregulated cocktail. A breathing tube had been inserted into her trachea and, astounding to recall, there was a person at her side manually inflating her lungs with an oxygen/air mixture. Day and night squeezing the bag with rates and pressures varying with the energy level of the person. What hope was there for this woman? The patient was suddenly restless and difficult to control. Another seizure occurred. And a fetal head was seen about to emerge. Blades of a simple pair of obstetric forceps were applied with the patient lying on her left side. A small but vigorous baby greeted all but her mother. Mother was still comatose. In the absence of imaging, a diagnosis of cerebral hemorrhage was made. Just a question of when to retire the bag squeezer.

An atonal poem it was. They all had eclampsia, their admission ticket. But none resembled the other. Renal shutdown in one, premature placental separation with loss of fetal life in another, fluid everywhere in a patient, making her unrecognizable. Even— her lungs were flooded—a near drowning.

And then there were just plain old fits. Wearily, privately, I thought: Couldn't they at least have the decency to seize in synchrony rather than at random? I pictured myself as the conductor of this awesome orchestra. Baton in hand, spatula, airway, oxygen, thorazine. But everything was chance and random with us stumbling from crisis to crisis with little control. 'Out of control' described my life in the eclampsia ward.

Coming out of the darkened ward squinting into the late afternoon African sunlight gave the disorienting feeling of coming out of a dark theater after a bad movie.

I had to continue with the actions of real life. Give rides, go home, cook, eat.

A sound, sound sleep and back again to this ward full of silence and secrets.

Ectopic gestation

She felt something give and then passed out. She worked as a maid in this Ob/Gyn doctor's house. He was a recent import from Britain with Missionary and Catholic written all over him. He and his family lived on 'the hill' in a wide solid colonial house and quickly slipped into the life. Maids, cooks, clubs. I lived that way, too, minus the clubs. One of the 'peaces' I discovered of living in the West was the pleasure of washing my own soiled clothes. It is false to excuse this master-and-servant way of life based on giving 'them' a job. That huge populace of household workers will find better ways if this unskilled, untrained, ill-paid outlet is cancelled. And it is joy not to depend on help and not have this help roaming around one's privacy.

Here she was, and it was not a difficult diagnosis. The incidence of ectopic gestation was 1 in 100, and we had a hundred deliveries a day. An ectopic a day to keep us in business. The patient was pale, anemic, hypotensive, but had a slow bounding pulse rate. The abdomen was distended, but soft as newly risen dough.

'Blood in the abdomen did not cause signs of peritoneal irritation': another one of Coralie's truths.

I was able to elicit 'shifting dullness.' Turning the patient to her side caused the dull-sounding blood to flow to the bottom and the air-filled gut to float on top to give a hollow-sounding note. Turn her to the other side and everything swished over again, thus the 'shifting dullness.'

Put it all together—anemic, hypotensive, shifting dullness because of a belly full of blood. No pregnancy tests or imaging to help and none needed. She had an ectopic gestation that had ruptured. The fertilized embryo had wandered down the Fallopian tube and instead of unimpeded passage to the plush and prepared uterus, it lost its way. Crevices and scars in the Fallopian tube, the result of partially healed previous infection, waylaid this little dot of love, and it implanted and started to grow in the thin-walled tube instead of the robust uterus. The mini-placenta secretes estrogens and progesterone to delude the uterus into thinking it is pregnant and it enlarges, often confusing the clinical diagnosis. The placenta, with the intensity of a burrowing mole, invades the flimsy tube, expands and distends it, and eventually erodes through a blood vessel. The blood flow through this area has been increased manyfold, and the blood vessel spills its pulsating content into the abdominal cavity. By the time shifting dullness is elicited, there are at least two liters of blood spilt.

We took her to the operating room fast. No need to wait for blood—there would be plenty of her own in the abdomen that could be salvaged and used. Waiting is the only mistake in this situation. Swift surgical correction the only answer.

Under general anesthesia we opened through a large vertical midline incision. Cosmetics were of no value to us. The diagnosis was confirmed just before opening the peritoneal layer which was discolored a give-away blue from the blood it held. Caution in the next step as we did not want to spill all this precious, best-matched blood. A small incision was made in the tented-up peritoneal layer to start collecting the patient's blood. Unbelievable, but the instruments used to collect the blood were a steel tablespoon and a ladle picked off someone's kitchen table. The blood was collected in a bowl, handed to a circulator who poured it via a funnel through several layers of gauze into a glass bottle containing a citrate anticoagulant. She handed the bottle to the anesthesiologist who poured it back into the patient.

There is a temptation to 'do a good job' collecting blood and use every corpuscle, but one has to stop at a reasonable point. The cause of the bleeding is still unattended. The peritoneal incision was extended—don't cry over spilt blood—there was loads of it. A hand into the pelvis lifted out the deluded uterus. Take a moment for a careful look. Sometimes back bleeding into the innocent tube makes it seem like the culprit. Examine both tubes before excising the injured one.

But this time both tubes appeared innocent. For pity's sake, this flood had to come from somewhere. And then we spied it. A tiny tongue of placental tissue protruding from the cornu of the uterus, the top right corner of the uterus where the right tube opened into it. A little nothing thing with blood gurgling out around it. A 'cornual' pregnancy, horrid because of the rapid blood loss and also because of the surgery it requires, which weakens the uterus at the tube junction. The tube and a generous chunk of uterus were removed and sutured over to stop the bleeding. Sutured and sutured to stop the bleeding. Surgical needles at the time had eyes and had to be threaded with catgut, literally made from some animal's gut. Because of the clumsiness of the suture material, each needle puncture bled independently and maddeningly. A dry closure was a feat of patience more than skill.

At the end of the surgery, I talked to the Ob/Gyn whose maid the patient was. I advised birth control to allow the uterus to heal. He bristled catholically. 'I don't believe in those things.'

He didn't believe in 'those things,' and I did not think to advise the patient directly—thought I had done my job by informing her unlikely guardian. I cringe at my arrogance.

NSVD in an iron lung

One of the hardest things for a young physician is to maintain some semblance of balance between living an ordinary life and then being plunged into extraordinary situations. I was planning a dinner party, the first in our new apartment and also the first ever as a married couple. A menu from my bible 'Time and Talents' cookbook, replete with misprints and coy quotations. The few friends we had outside the Tejani clan were invited, and we were personally affronted if some said they could not make it. I remember we wavered and changed the date several times so that everyone we asked could come. What could be so satisfying about having some people over, producing a meal, talking of extraordinary mundanenesses. And yet I remember the glow after it was over. And then it was all forgotten when the next day I met her.

At first I met her head only. The rest of her was in this fiberglass and metal case. Her body appeared in waves of distortion because of the vagaries in throw and measure of the glass through which it was viewed. Who was this head sealed off from the rest of her young body? She was unable to speak because her breathing was dictated by the contraption she was attached to. Light black and painfully young was she.

She had been brought by taxi the night before from her village. Her family reported weakness in her legs for a few days, and then the previous evening she grew restless and appeared to have difficulty breathing. A neighbor's friend was a taxi driver and agreed to take her to a local clinic, a distance of twenty miles. There they identified polio, and the taxi brought her the additional forty miles to the country's only University Hospital.

Admitted through the Emergency Room, she had progressive difficulty breathing, and her efforts became shallow and ineffective. She was thought to have the dreaded 'ascending' poliomyelitis and was brought to this room in an isolated building adjoining the hospital. Where a respirator would have been used today, she was entered into this fiberglass and steel case, a 'coffin on wheels.' A pair of bellows periodically reduced the pressure of air surrounding the patient, causing her lungs to expand and take in room air. Release of the negative pressure made her exhale.

Oh, and by the way, she was eight months pregnant with her first baby.

To allow access to the patient, there were two rotating ports on the right side of the 'iron lung.' When opened, they led to canvas sleeves ending in enormous gloves—one size for all—through which we entered our arms and hands for access to the patient. The examination process had to be rapid as the seal and therefore the respiratory assistance was partially lost during this maneuver. From the corner of my eyes I saw other ports without sleeves. Made a mental note of them for the dreaded anticipated delivery.

How to assess this patient? Back to basics—physical examination is inspection, palpation, percussion and auscultation--observing, feeling and hearing what one could. Auscultation was the only step that required the help of a stethoscope. The rest was done using eyes and hands. Inspection through the distorted fiberglass lid revealed a possibly pregnant abdomen, more convincing now that I was told she was pregnant. Palpation next. I nervously undid the ports and rapidly felt her abdomen through the rough canvas sleeves and gloves fashioned for the giant Abbi-Yoyo. I could just make out a fetal head in the lower pole of the uterus. Reassuring. Any other presentation would have added layers of problems. In the days before sonography our clinical findings were actually reliable. No question of auscultation for the fetal heartbeat. I tried without success to apply a stethoscope to her belly through the clumsy unyielding sleeve. When asked if the baby moved, she nodded with dark eyes filled with something beyond fear.

A madcap Professor Heyns from South Africa had written extensively on the advantages of applying negative pressure to the pregnant woman's abdomen. In my mind, anything from South Africa was suspect in those apartheid days. He wrote that pain in labor was due to pressure of the contracting uterus on the abdominal wall. Negative pressure applied through his space suit would raise the abdominal wall from the uterus and prevent pain. He claimed that it also improved the efficiency of the contraction, thus expediting labor. He then went on flights of fancy and declared that if applied during pregnancy, it enhanced fetal growth as the negative pressure opened up blood vessels and thus enhanced blood flow to the uterus. He further defied sanity by using a negative pressure device over the vaginal opening to facilitate delivery and—crowning glory—shorten the time to the delivery of the placenta. His work was bolstered by conviction and never burdened with control groups. Evidence-based medicine was for anti-apartheid skeptics.

Professor Heyns was with me in spirit when it was time to deliver her.

A few nights later, when she was about 34 weeks pregnant, she changed from her usual calmness to an uneasiness and then a restlessness that could not be controlled by her nurse's soothings. Ever sensitive to the moods of her silent patient, the nurse was sure that some new development was occurring.

Her restlessness was periodic—every five minutes. Between, she was quiet, even asleep. It could only be labor. Now what? I, we, waited a few hours. During this time, I realized that Professor Heyns was right. Every time a contraction would coincide with a negative pressure induction, she would be calm, as the Professor had predicted. The negative pressure drawing the abdomen away from the uterus gave her the relief she needed.

As the contractions came closer and stronger, we temporarily opened a port for a vaginal examination. She was fully dilated. Heyns was right again. Her first stage had lasted only four hours. Negative pressure expedited labor!

We noted that she did not do well during the discontinuation of respiratory assistance, even for the brief pelvic examination. She was distressed and blue after the ordeal. She could not possibly be disconnected long enough for delivery.

The fumbling decision of how to deliver her was taken out of our hands as we saw the perineum bulge with each contraction. Again the best progress was made when the negative pressure coincided with a contraction. We discussed whether we could time the iron-lung pressure cycles to coincide with contractions. Such flexibility was not to be, but just increasing the rate captured more of the contractions.

Thoughts on her delivery. Visions of blood and amniotic fluid flung everywhere in her glass case, if caught at a negative pressure phase. Delivery in a weightless environment could be an awful mess. Imagine a delivery in a spaceship. Containment had to be the answer. We slipped in a sheet to isolate the perineum from the rest of her and watched transfixed as the birth process unfolded rapidly and efficiently with no help from her attendants. Women deliver babies, not obstetricians.

We watched through the distorted glass as the baby's head smoothly crowned and then delivered itself by a process of extending the up-to-now flexed head. It then restituted—untwisting its neck toward the mother's right side—continued this movement—external rotation till it faced the mother's left thigh. A moment later, a grunt and the anterior and then the posterior shoulder came into view. Slippery-slided out a perfect baby. Quick hands clamped the cord and delivered the little thing through the open port. Full marks on the Apgar score, top of the class. We continued to observe as the placenta delivered rapidly, aided in its journey by negative pressure episodes. Almost no bleeding occurred after the placenta was delivered. A neat clean lovely delivery. That euphemistic NSVD—normal spontaneous vaginal delivery—in an iron lung, no less. I was by now a firm Heyns-ite.

The best was yet to come. The next few days showed her less dependent on respiratory assistance. And in a week she was delivered from her 'coffin on wheels.' There was no escaping that her recovery started with that magnificent delivery. An obstetrician's firm religion is that pregnancy neither makes worse nor better any coincidental maternal disorder. Her recovery could have been coincidence, or maybe there are flaws in our religious beliefs.

She went home with minimal weakness in her right leg. She went home breast-feeding and smiling. Before she left, she requested to see her iron lung again. And bid it sweet goodbye.

Unspeakable deeds

When I first came to the U.S. in 1971, I realized there was an etiquette for physicians trained in other countries to follow when retraining. This involved suppression of previous experiences lest they sound out of tune with local mores. To develop a smile that betrayed neither superiority nor gaps in one's knowledge. A fellow immigrant called this 'a gesture life.' No matter, our children will be the participators. As years roll on and some credibility is established, some experiences leak. If smartly timed, they are well received.

There are some, however, that always remain unspeakable: difficult to recount to fellow obstetricians and impossible to confess to my children.

Obstetric destructive procedures were widely used in the Africa of the '60s. Women laboring in the villages for long hours, often days, would be brought in exhausted, infected, with the fetus long dead, amniotic fluid lost and the uterus tightly spread over the little corpse, thinned out and on the verge of rupture. Any internal maneuver would be the ultimate catstrophe for this depleted patient. Any maneuver without reducing the bulk of the uterine contents would cause this fragile uterus to rupture. To the rescue — the obstetric destructive procedures.

She had been in labor for several days and nights. Much had been tried by the village women, including a dark leafy poultice that filled her vagina and covered the little arm and perfect fingers that protruded from her vagina. The fetal heartbeat had long given up—silent. A tube was inserted to empty the mother's stomach prior to anticipated general anesthesia. Out poured an evil green fluid full of fragments of leaf and bark. *Dagara Kiganda*, this stuff was called, 'medicine of the Kiganda tribe.' Its effect was to cause explosive unregulated uterine contractions. The tree used was a secret unavailable to any but the local witches. It is difficult to believe that no one investigated this possibly useful medication. Arrogance, again, played a large part in our daily lives. We had pitocin, and this ancient remedy was cast off as evil and not to be contemplated. Without a doubt where conditions were right, many unseen women delivered expeditiously because of it.

But conditions were not right here. There was an impasse with the fetus lying transversely, the uterus stretched into a Valentine's day heart shape with the fetal head on the right and the breech on the left. And the give-away little arm dipping into and protruding from the vagina.

The options were a cesarean section for this already dead baby on an exhausted dehydrated infected woman. If she had come in earlier with more amniotic fluid, the fetus could be turned and delivered as a breech birth. But this procedure in such a long-neglected patient would certainly cause the ultimate catastrophe of a ruptured uterus. So we proceded to—call it by its real name—decapitation. Horrendous to think of, but life-saving for the patient.

Deep general anesthesia was used for relaxation and maneuverability, but also as a good solution for oblivion—who could tell the patient what went on? Traction on the little arm brought the fetal neck within reach. Ready for this? The decapitation instrument, a hook-shaped knife, was inserted beyond and then rotated to lie across the fetal neck. Once this was accomplished an up-and-down sawing was started. To keep thoughts at a distance and relieve fatigue, a tune would go through my mind—sawing in time to 'Waltzing Matilda.' I've never been able to tolerate that song since. Tender tissues are cut through and the last part aided with scissors. When separated, the torso was delivered easily and the tissues of the neck presented. These were grasped with tissue forceps and the head delivered as the after-coming head of a breech birth—only...the mother woke up. Although she knew the baby was lost, she wanted to see it. Dear nurses pieced it together and asked me to put in a few stitches to prevent the head from wobbling. They arranged blankets strategically to smother the event. Mother was sad but did not seem to notice the results of what went on while she was oblivious.

Humans adjust, forgive and move on.

From Caesar's time

Dr. Jim Jones, the chairman I worked with in the '90s, gave me a slide of an ancient woodcut. It shows two angels delivering a bonny baby from an oblivious woman. The baby is emerging from a generous vertical incision in the mother's belly. Nearby stands a haloed Mary-like woman observing the birth. Dr. Jones' interpretation was that the angels were early fellows in training performing a cesarean section under the supervision of Mary, the perinatologist. I think it is a post-mortem cesarean section with the mother clearly dead and in the hands of the angels. The world of angels was not ready for the baby.

She came in from the *charo* three days in labor, 'ready to deliver' for all of one day. Most ominously, we were told that 'everything' had

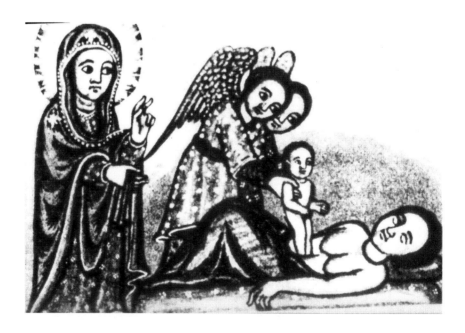

been done. Everything usually included the same *dagara kiganda*, an herbal brew from the leaves and bark of that secret tree that caused violent uterine contractions that either expedited delivery or, in an impasse, ruptured the uterus. The woman was exhausted, but there was still a fetal heartbeat. The uterus was hourglass-shaped and wrapped closely around the fetus. The lower part was distended, and any false move would cause its rupture. There was still hope with hydration, antibiotics and a cesarean section.

We took her to the operating rooms, and the anesthesiologist prepared her for general anesthesia. Seconds after induction, as the anesthesiologist fumbled for the endotracheal tube, the patient gave a mighty heave and brought up macerated leaves and small pieces of bark in a dark soup. Then, before our eyes, she inhaled and I could almost see the evil fluid enter her larynx, trachea, bronchi, bronchioles and the ultimate spaces where oxygen is exchanged. She was momentarily agitated and restless and then fell deathly quiet.

What had been the reason for the ancient Caesarean law to deliver women who died in late pregnancy by cutting out the baby? Did large numbers of women die in late pregnancy? I came back to earth. I realized that this was what was expected of me. The consultant had told me on the phone call which I had made before this catastrophe had occurred, to start surgery and she would be in presently. She was nowhere in sight.

In many ways, this was the perfect set-up for this catastrophe. In the operating room, a scrubbed surgeon, instruments, assistant, anesthesiologist were all at hand. I realized that speed was everything. I had read that a vertical single slash through the skin, fat, fascia, peritoneum, uterine wall and amniotic membranes should reach the baby in seconds and the fetus would be rescued. It was atrociously difficult to go against the grain. Layers, careful layers, I had always been taught. My trembling hands did not help matters. I should have remembered the old adage that often brings courage: 'Can't make things any worse than they are.'

The patient had been dead for at least five minutes before this otherwise perfect baby was born. Those angel fellows in training must have helped because there was a heartbeat. A heartbeat is hope. A tiny tube was slipped into the baby's trachea and the nice compliant lungs were inflated with an air/oxygen mixture. The heart rate picked up but the baby remained unresponsive. We took turns inflating the bag all night. What were we thinking? Where would this motherless compromised baby go? Pure desperation guided us.

Morning brought common sense and the consultant required us to desist and go back to real work.

Goodbye.

Nationality

There is something about that slim book, blue, black, green, blood-colored, encrusted with the country you are supposed to be devoted to. Primary immigrants have a certain look when they present a U.S. passport to surly customs officers. Proud at first when they avoid the ragged 'non-U.S. citizen' lines, but so nervous—as though one misstep would cause the document to revert to some inferior form. I am happy that I did not get attached to my passport, because I had more of them than Elizabeth Taylor had husbands.

I was born in India during the British Raj—therefore British to start with. After Independence and the euphoria of midnight August 15th, 1948, we exchanged the relic of the Raj for Indian passports complete with lions and the Chakra, ancient symbol of the great king Ashoka. On arrival in Uganda, my medical registration, registrar's job and subsequent commonwealth scholarship were favored by a British passport. So in 1960 back to British became I. Later, in 1962, Ugandan independence resulted in euphoria number two and I sported a Ugandan Crested Crane on my passport. In 1971, with the Crested Crane, I flew to New York. A year later, in 1972, with the Asians being removed from Uganda by Idi Amin, the result of his divine dream, I and we had no papers. Stateless and free were we. Quite free, but not free to travel, though we did, with some scraps of paper declaring who we were. During this time, I received, in New York, a bedraggled letter from the Government of Uganda, advising me that I was not required to leave even though I had committed the crime of being brown (my cynicism). He called upon my altruism and reminded me that I could serve my country since I was a doctor. The letter was signed by Idi Amin. Unlike vicious rumor, he did not apply a thumbprint, but his full name and flourish. Needless to say at that point, we declined the invitation.

Following this, in 1976, Amir and I became U.S. citizens and have been ever since. Many around me say they have a sentimental spiritual genetic attachment to the nationality of their birth or original country of emigration. We rationalized our fickleness by saying we belonged to the country that gives us our bread.

And yet eons ago, as a schoolgirl in Bombay at the Alexandra High School for Girls, from a slim volume entitled 'Poets and Poetry,' I was required to memorize poems, many quite evocative, of English poets expressing their love of country: 'Some corner of a foreign field / That is forever England.'

And even more, although I cannot remember when it was first imprinted in memory,

> ...this scept'red isle,
> This other Eden, demi-paradise,
> This fortress built by Nature for herself
> Against infection and the hand of war...
> This precious stone set in the silver sea...
> This blessed plot, this earth, this realm, this England...
> This land of such dear souls, this dear dear land...

I am envious of those who have this feeling of belonging. And yet I cannot imagine what my life and loves would have been if all had to be shared with my adoration of country. 'No room, no room,' as the Mad Hatter said to Alice.

And there I was, brown, living in Uganda, British again and, strange to ponder, one who had never set foot on that scept'red isle.

The case of the jackfruit

All Ugandan *shambas*, even the smallest gardens, grew local fruits. Papayas, mindful of always having a male tree to fertilize the fruiting females, avocado, the small sun-yellow sweetest-of-sweet Uganda pineapples. Of all the tropical fruit, jackfruit is the strangest. Growing on tall trees usually wild in forests, the fruit grows straight off the bark of the tree and is large, warty and boggy to feel. The meat has a certain over-ripe smell even when fresh, and the fibrous consistence and taste is meaty. A non-vegetarian fruit.

The pernicious habit of using items of food to describe pathology is universal—grapefruit-, lemon- or orange-sized. Citrus is definitely favored. But here is the story of a jackfruit.

This was her first baby. She was brought in by her sister, who was also the village midwife. The midwife had once worked for a short while in the maternity ward of an area hospital and was bright and talkative.

'Something is not right,' she said. Labor had lasted a day, and she had been fully dilated for several hours, but the fetal head remained high and would not descend into the pelvis.

'And,' she said, 'instead of the fetal head feeling like a coconut, it feels like a jackfruit.'

I examined the tired woman. The lower part of her uterus was tender and occupied by a soft large mass which did not feel like a fetal head. A breech presentation? But the baby's bottom was clearly felt in the usual place, high under the mother's rib cage. A pelvic examination confirmed full dilatation and the jackfruit high up. Wide-open boggy-feeling fontanels and sutures. This had to be fetal hydrocephalus—a ballooning of the brain with cerebrospinal fluid because of an obstruction preventing its egress and absorption. My consultant, Dr. Daphne Kayton, who later delivered my firstborn, agreed with this diagnosis.

What to do? The already thinned-out lower uterus was in danger of rupture. A cesarean section was an option of last resort, firstly because circumstance and distance might not allow this woman to return to hospital in another pregnancy. Also, this would result in the live birth of this inevitably compromised baby in this country where even the fittest infants have trouble staying alive. A major surgical procedure resulting in a handicapped child was unacceptable to patient and sister.

The alternative was to drain the fluid through a needle passed into the ballooned brain. This would cause the skull to collapse, accommodating it for vaginal delivery. And it would likely result in a dead birth without the wrenching decisions on how to deal with this doomed baby.

But what if our diagnosis was not correct? A needle in a normal brain. Too terrible to contemplate. The patient's voice aroused me from my dithering. She had had enough and had not made this journey for talk and indecision. Her sister had already made the diagnosis—now action, please.

We took her to the operating room. I felt my misgivings in my heart, which had suddenly decided to make its presence felt. What if? Dr. Kayton is calm and easy. Years of experience make her say, 'We'll soon find out.'

The patient is positioned for the procedure. Go ahead. Take that twenty-gauge long spinal needle. Protect the vaginal walls with your own fingers as it is introduced and guide it up to the jackfruit head. Then do it.

Relief of dearest reliefs. Out poured a fountain of crystal clear spring water, spewing its size away. My grateful hands hold the needle in place as I feel the compliant head gradually take the shape of the pelvis and enter its pelvic journey. 'Don't forget the last step,' says Dr. Kayton. She wants me to push and turn the needle in deeper so as to ensure a dead baby. I do this with ease. I understand and sympathize with this step very well. It sits perfectly well with me.

A few contractions, a mother's grunt, and this perfect face with a deflated balloon head was in my hands. Slippery eel body followed. Further relief—no sign of life.

Dr. Kayton and I stand on the grassy verge outside the operating room. She had her inevitable cigarette between her lips and was making plans for the weekend. A trip to Murchison Falls with a visiting Brit.

This spectacular sad country.

The year ends

The training year was ending. My book, the blue and gold tome, was close to complete. Professor Coralie called me to say that I should spend some time in British teaching hospitals to learn things pertinent to the MRCOG examination. How long? Nine months, forty weeks, like a pregnancy. How were we ever going to afford this? She looked surprised, as she thought all Indians had to have silent money stowed away. 'No,' I said, 'I'm serious.'

Being a woman with unlimited resources, without any hesitation, she went to plan B. The British Commonwealth Scholarship committee awarded scholarships every year to deserving 'natives' for higher studies in the U.K. The understanding was that the 'native' would then return and pay back in kind to the country of origin. She quite frankly warned me that I did not look like a Ugandan native, which might be a problem.

She provided me with all the needed paperwork, which was neatly filled in by Amir as I am congenitally unable to fill in forms. I never saw it, but she must have written an excellent letter for me. I had to ask two others to write letters as well. I carefully avoided Dr. Crabby G and asked Professor Williams and Dr. Kayton to write on my behalf.

I was asked to come for an interview, and I remember a giant half circle of formidable males with me, sitting, confronting them. But they seemed unusually friendly and jovial. Toward the end of a twenty-minute session, I realized they had decided in my favor way before I had entered the room. I realized Professor Coralie Rendle-Short had already spoken for me and won this bristly group over.

I soon received a letter congratulating me and cordially wishing me a happy and profitable stay in Britain. This warm letter was signed by an individual who called himself 'Scarborough.' A hereditary Lord or Earl of some sort with single-name recognition like Madonna or Cher. I would surely have stuttered and stumbled if I had known that single-named Scarborough was amongst the formidable males I had faced at the interview.

Coralie congratulated me before I had heard from Scarborough. She helped me get into Charing Cross Hospital as an observer for four months, which time would also include two weeks at Jessop Hospital in Sheffield to observe surgery for pelvic relaxation and stress incontinence which I had no exposure to in Uganda (remember that backward pelvic tilt that keeps weight off the pelvic floor). After that she recommended a four-month course based at Queen Charlotte's Hospital specially designed toward the MRCOG examination. The last of my nine months would be spent in written and oral exam-taking and waiting for the results since I could not afford to return if I did not pass.

It is somewhat dismaying to relate what I learned in that intense, sleepless, physically and mentally taxing year to my subsequent obstetric practice. Close to nothing lay in common. But maybe that is not the purpose of good training. Perhaps the important things that Coralie and Professor Williams and the host of others taught me were habits and not techniques, universally and forever applicable. Habits, you see. The habit of reading. The habit of why, why, why. The habit of loving that dear pregnant woman. The habit of using every action to teach younger people in the field. If this smells of naiveté, so be it. It has enabled me to live well.

The prospect of leaving and separation for nine months suddenly lay heavy on Amir and me. It became a reality with the news that I had been awarded the scholarship. Passage to and back, payment for the courses, a book and clothing allowance and fifty pounds a month to live on. More than generous. More than I had ever earned before in my life. Daphne (Kayton) said it was going to be cold when I got there. So we went to the only local department store in Kampala, Deacon's, and bought a brown jersey skirt and jacket with pseudo leather trim labeled 'Marks and Spencer.' K, my Nairobi cousin JL's unhappy wife, commented that my maid would be wearing the same. Since I was unlikely to have contact with any maids, I did not see that as a problem. We had stopped at Nairobi on our drive down to Mombasa, a farewell trip. As usual we made a round of the Nairobi National Park. Goodbye, gazelles, goodbye. Miss me if you can. This time we also stopped at Tsavo and watched the gentle quiet elephants, mothers and children, aunts and grandmothers, all in patient play.

A honeymoon it was. We stayed at the Oceanic Hotel in Mombasa and swam and loved the short week away. Amir's cousin, the first family member to greet me in Africa, now ran a hotel and restaurant in Malindi near Mombasa. He gave us *samosas* to picnic with on the snowy white Malindi beaches, but charged us for lunch.

THREE

Nine Months in London

1962: Nine months in London

We gave up our cozy blue apartment, and Amir moved back with his mother, and one lonely November night in 1961, I flew away in my Marks and Spencer suit. A cold desolation on the plane and even worse on landing at Heathrow—a foggy dark London dawn. A representative of the scholarship committee met me and drove me to the British Commonwealth hostel. She gave me a list of rooming possibilities and my first month's installment of fifty pounds and some more for clothing. That afternoon I went to the hostel cafeteria and stood in line for lunch. I almost choked when I saw a giant piece of overcooked meat on the recognizable femur of some poor cow.

I avoided the cow and sat down with some potatoes, and suddenly heard my name. Coming over to me was yet another Tejani cousin, Roshan. She was smiling and sweet, had been there a few days, and knew of my arrival. Having lived in London before, she knew her way around.

She wolfed down the cow lunch —'free food,' she said heartily. After she had finished, she took me via the underground to Oxford Street and, so that I wouldn't be wearing the same clothes as my maid, and since I had fifty-plus pounds in my pocket, I bought a tweedy-looking warm coat with a giant knitted collar from Selfridge's that served me well through the soon-to-come winter. Some skirts and sweaters later, we returned, and suddenly the bustle and lights of a big city seemed fun and warming.

I quickly mastered the London tubes—very different from the

complicated New York subway, which took me years to understand. The next day I went to Clapham Common and walked to the address given to me. The landlady was impossibly old but welcoming and gave me one of those crippling gripping British handshakes which I slowly developed a technique for anticipating and steeling myself to prevent injury. She showed me into a pleasant flowery bedroom and living and dining rooms that I could use. I was to share the bathroom with a portly-looking German student. Included in the rent was breakfast and dinner, which the poor woman was to prepare for her lodgers. I saw nothing wrong with it and brought my luggage over in a taxi.

I noticed that the landlady did not invite me into the kitchen, in fact, told me it was off bounds. She would firmly refuse when I, as I had been instructed to, offered help with the cooking or doing the dishes. Just as well, thought I, never having washed a dish in my life, though the firmness with which she turned me away from the kitchen was eerie. I couldn't help thinking that some weird thing was locked up in the kitchen.

My landlady was at her best in the morning when she would tell me and the portly German what she intended to cook for dinner. Wonderful dishes of roast meats, green and yellow vegetables, roast potatoes, Yorkshire pudding, and as her mouth watered she'd say 'parsnips.' When dinnertime rolled around, all would be forgotten, and there would be a piece of indeterminate meat and some gray mush.

I started work at Charing Cross Hospital and soon discovered that an observer's position, after the kind of year I had just experienced, was impossibly boring. I filled a few hours each day in the clinics, private offices and operating rooms of the consultants and then slowly discovered the allure of London. Prime amongst them was Charing Cross Road with its row of used and rare book stores. Every time I have been to London since, this has been my favorite haunt.

An unforgettable no-nonsense person I met was Dr. Josephine Barnes, who, once a week, would take me down to a country hospital where she operated. She was lean and mean and efficient. Had an answer for everything and time for nothing. Her brother was an internist with a special interest in obstetrics and had written a book on medical disorders in pregnancy — the first of its kind with many authors later following his lead.

A distant aunt of mine, later a food writer, lived in London at this time and often invited me over for her rather trendy soirees. She would invite a balanced and carefully thought-out group and 'entertain' with a capital E. Nothing momentous ever happened at these gatherings. I often went with an old Parsi eccentric who lived near me. Jal Tata saw and lived with ghosts and often spoke of a lady in white who routinely crept in at night and sat chatting on his bed. He was a confirmed bachelor, I think it was wishful thinking. He would meet me, sockless, near a tube station, and we would travel together, all the while talking of the supernatural. At my Aunt B's home, he would take his hat off. In his hat were a rolled-up pair of socks 'all nice and warm.' He would don them in preparation for the evening's fun.

One day Aunt A had on her special British accent for some English fawner whose qualification was that he had briefly been in India. The two of them went on and on about the deterioration, rudeness and unreliability of help, servants, slaves in India. After half an hour of this, I could take it no more and left, unfortunately unfed. I wandered into a movie house and saw that darling Audrey Hepburn as Holly Golitely in Truman Capote's 'Breakfast at Tiffany's.' 'Moon River' always brings me back to the day I gave up A's comforts for what? Only after I came to the U.S. thirty years later did I discover that I hated the institution of domestic help and found a freedom in the substandard state of my private home.

Having burnt my bridges with A, I spent more time with Laila, Amir's sister, who had come to London from Kampala the year before. She had worked at the UEB, the Uganda Electricity Board, and its chief, Erisa Kironde, had given her a scholarship to learn ways of promoting electricity over the use of coal and wood-standards in Uganda. She lived with her now life-long friend Zarin in a one-room apartment with a kitchen at the far end where she made comfort meals for all of us. She was in love, and it showed. Her normally pretty face glowed with that extra magic. She had met a young man in London, and the four of us had good times together with cheap wine, music and walks in the park.

A week at Jessop Hospital in Sheffield also in the dubious

observer role did not help much, though I did learn the theoretic basics of pelvic floor repair from discontented, sneering senior registrars. The bottle-neck at the senior registrar level was all-pervasive, and this malcontent group waited around, grudgingly doing the job, hoping for the death of one of the consultants so as to create a position. If they ever talked to me, it was to assure me repeatedly that an African experience had no relationship to passing the MRCOG examination.

I returned to Clapham Common from Sheffield one afternoon and, to announce my presence, entered the landlady's forbidden kitchen. She sat at the kitchen table with her head resting on her arms, with several empty bottles of Guinness at her elbow. Piled high in the sink and on the floor and almost everywhere else there were dirty dishes with congealing fat and food. She opened her eyes as I entered and had a fit of anger, reminding me how I was not supposed to enter the kitchen.

I resolved to leave this unhappy woman's world, and my contact at the British Commonwealth office gave me an address in Ealing. This was a hostel run by Catholic nuns. I took it sight unseen and bid the strange woman goodbye.

The convent hostel had pleasant but underheated rooms, common dining times with fine food in small portions, and rosy-cheeked smiling nuns all playing at being children before the Mother Superior. One day Mother Superior called me to her office and took me to a room where she introduced me to a sullen-faced teenaged Irish girl. She asked me to examine her abdomen, which was unquestionably 18-20 weeks pregnant. There followed a recriminatory though forgiving sermon to the girl, who was to be sent to a home for 'wayward girls' the next day. I gathered that I was to accompany her to give the information of her pregnancy to the 'wayward' keepers.

That night at dinner, the Irish girl sat at a table next to mine. Suddenly, halfway through dinner, she started a loud steady stream of curses and obscenities toward the Catholic system and everything else that had battered her young life. A middle-aged woman who held daily court at one of the other tables broke the spell and threw her napkin down and said she would not hear this slander anymore. An insistent group of black-habited penguin nuns surrounded the rebellious lass, and she suddenly crumpled and allowed herself to be led from the room. In the end, she was Catholic, and was impressed by the enormity of her sin.

The next day I met Mother Superior and a solid bald fast-talking ingratiating lawyer whom Mother was obviously dependent upon. His passport to heaven was the *pro bono* work he did for these nuns. He drove us to the wayward home where I declared her to be pregnant to the attendants. And she was soon folded into a system of which I had no understanding. I left with the balding lawyer, regretting that I had not been a better advocate for the girl. No matter. She was probably getting the care that she understood best. Her child must now be forty years old.

London: Bright lights

As I was preparing to leave the nunnery in early February 1962 to start the course at Queen Charlotte's Hospital I got a call from my co-trainee in Uganda, Gareth Barberton. He had flown out from Africa on his birthday and moved into Queen Charlotte's Hostel, preparatory to the course we had been booked into. Hello and can we meet? We met the next day at pigeon-contaminated Nelson's feet, near the southeastern lion—the one that stares (stonily) at Africa.

A few days later I moved into a room at the Queen Charlotte's Dormitory. Two rows of single small basic rooms with a bathroom to each row. The others at the course were a group of raucous beer-guzzling Australians (one morning I crashed into a Giza-high pyramid of beer bottles they had piled outside my door—this was as subtle as their jokes could get), a passionate, hot Iranian with a stream of flashy girlfriends, a huddled-together mostly female sari-wearing group from India and an Englishman who looked like a rough tough soccer player, but talked only of *Der Rosenkavalier*, and who was obviously having difficulty passing the boards.

Then there were two people who had no intention of appearing for the boards, but were just relaxing at the course. One, a big blond Aryan-looking Israeli, LK, amused us all with an adage or irony for every situation. I heard that he became an autocratic, dictatorial chairman at Kaplan Hospital in Rehovat, Israel. Years later, I met him at a perinatal meeting in the U.S. Recharging his batteries, he said with his old twinkle. But otherwise, age and circumstance had made him lose his shine and increase his bulk. I remember him mock-complaining of his wife Schiffra, whom he obviously adored. *Schiffra* meant a grain of wheat, he told me. I made a note of this lovely name for future use.

The second non-exam-taker was Siu Fun, a fortyish Chinese woman from Hong Kong. In Hong Kong her home was on the elitist 'hill' where the richest people lived. Here, however, she had been doing serial *locum tenens* jobs in search of eventually doing her MRCOG. She had just ended a love affair with a man twenty years her junior. But more about her later.

Also at the course, though not staying at Charlotte's, was a pregnant Zarina Chinchinwalla (nee Bibiji) who graduated from my medical school in India a year before me and married the class valedictorian, genius, and grand sweep prize-winner…much as Amir had done the following year.

The operatic Englishman, and later Gareth, had cars and would load as many as possible of the group to get to our various study sites. At Hammersmith Hospital, we made rounds with no less than Professor McLure Brown, who, we were deluded into believing, knew the cause of preeclampsia (it remains unknown to this day). His retinue was huge with the poor post-graduates attached to the tail end of the crowd. It was full of inside jokes and asides that somehow did not reach or impress me at the periphery. I remembered Professor Williams and his quiet introverted teaching.

In March, I received a royal-looking envelope—an invitation from Queen Elizabeth to a reception for all the commonwealth scholars. At first I thought it crude to accept hospitality from the person and the institution about whom I had such persistently negative thoughts. But the temptation was too much and I went. Armed with the invitation we were allowed past the babushka guards at the gates of Buckingham Palace and walked across the huge courtyard into an anteroom where there were at least a hundred other scholars. At some appointed time, the doors to an ornate room opened, and we helped ourselves to a rough-tasting sherry, hot eats that were lumpy and stone cold and cold ones that were lukewarm. I wandered around till I saw all eyes turn toward a door through which entered the queen, this ultra-diminutive woman with an unchanging smile and her tall smiling husband, Philip of Greece.

The scholars lined up to be introduced to the royal couple. A variety of gestures—curtsies, bows, namastes, and hand-shakes. The Queen, all the while with her bland smile, and Philip with a light comment for each person. When I got back I met Gareth. He was genuinely pleased that I had been so honored, but told me I was inappropriately dressed. I had worn an exquisite pinky-purple heavy silk sari, the color of the East African lilac-breasted roller. He said the next time I was invited (!) I should wear a dark suit, pearls, white gloves and a hat! I looked to see if he was teasing but he was not. As Frank Sinatra warbled in the middle of crooning 'A foggy day...' at the London Palladium also in 1962, 'an Englishman loves his queen.'

At Charlotte's, our principal teacher was Carl Wood, a tall rugged young Australian who had a style and energy that engulfed all. He was friendly with Gareth and me, and would often stay on after his talk to probe us about Africa. Later he published many memorable papers from Monash University about fetal acid-base status and later yet, assisted reproductive technologies. I have not seen him in the journals of late. I can never think of him as old—as he surely must be.

The book learning was easy enough. And spring came. I had only seen daffodils in Wordsworth before this spring. Daffodils have a certain spring scent. To my tropical eyes an English spring was astonishing. My first time with blossoming trees, peonies, lilac and tulips. All so gentle compared to our tropical flash. And the lime-colored new leaves. The two Ugandans went everywhere— museums, art galleries, the ballet at Covent Garden, shows and music, wonderful music. Menuhin at the Royal Festival Hall— Dubonnet and a twist in hand. One day at Gareth's alma mater, Oxford, we stood near an old grave marked February 29th in a year that could not have been a leap year since it was not divisible by four. And once, through the grass at Arundel, we heard and then saw Judy Garland emoting and entertaining her adoring retinue. And white moonlight on the ancient Thames.

The course ended and people left, Gareth to a cottage he had rented just outside London, a temporary shelter for him, his wife, Pat, and his three children, who had just wound things up in Uganda and flown over.

I next saw Gareth the day of the written examination. I finished early and wandered around the college. Tucked away in a corner were the original Chamberlain obstetric forceps—beautifully crafted in wood with the blades tied together with a length of what looked like hide. They had a perfect cephalic curve to accommodate the fetal head, but no pelvic curve to fit the mother's pelvis. I remembered the notorious story of the forceps being a secret, and when pressed to reveal his success, Chamberlain displayed only one blade, leaving people mystified.

My oral examination was scheduled a few days later. The obstetric case was a patient with twins who kindly helped me find both fetal heads and fetal heartbeats. My gynecologic patient was a woman with large fibroids. Fibroids were the bread and butter of practice in Uganda, and there could not be any aspect I was unfamiliar with. The Sheffield registrars' dire predictions of fumbling on pelvic relaxation never happened. These seasoned examiners seemed intent on discovering what I did know and not what I didn't. After the morning's cases, I went to an Indian restaurant and had a giant meal. My memory even seems to conjure up a glass of red wine.

I hope I brushed my teeth before I went to the college for the afternoon session where my cases were to be discussed and my two commentaries defended. But it went easily, with the examiners particularly interested in my gynecologic commentary on complications after abdominally performed gynecologic surgery. They advised me to shorten it and get it published, which I eventually did in the *East African Medical Journal*. I could have been more ambitious, but felt this was the patriotic thing to do. This was my very first publication, and I regret that I do not have a copy of it.

A few days later, Gareth visited me at the Charlotte's Hostel, having completed his oral exam. We talked for a while and then said *Kwaheri*, goodbye. We wished each other a good life, a wish that we took seriously and accomplished. And, with a wave, he drove away in his dark blue station wagon.

Then followed a period of waiting for the results. I was lonely and wrote Amir every day and he wrote back, sometimes two letters in a day. Amir had a unique style of writing, and amongst the possessions I have accumulated over the years, I cannot believe I have none of his letters. I love reading and rereading letters, and they would have served me well today. He used capitals in an unorthodox way, emphasizing a word, a syllable or sometimes whole paragraphs. He punned and joked and invented names for me. Invented words never heard before or since and always laughed and loved and laughed.

And my Chinese friend Sui Fun took me into her capable hands. The good woman stayed this extra time only to be with me. She regaled me with graphic accounts of her love affair with a man much younger than herself. Her Catholic machinations at birth control were especially funny. And we exchanged recipes. I gave her the recipe for roasted *nsenene*—grasshoppers. And she taught me how to make snake soup. She insisted I write down the steps, an unnecessary precaution, as I was unlikely to forget so unique a recipe. I was also unlikely to prepare this delicacy, especially since the first step was to capture the snake, grip it in a way to hold the mouth open, make a slit in the skin below its jaw and strip the skin off while the reptile was still alive—and then plunge the writhing naked body in boiling broth. And she thought the grasshopper recipe was equally rude and inedible!

Sui Fun and I took a trip up to Hampstead Heath to hear Sibelius' Second Symphony. A glorious evening, lying in the park on a hill with the orchestra at the bottom of the hill, and a small lake just beyond. She bought the LP vinyl record for me and inscribed it in that language which was all her own. I listened to it recently and, apart from a few hiccups, it was perfect. She dated it August 2nd 1962 and wrote 'My dear Nergesh, Very be careful of this record that we both like.' After I had my first baby girl, she sent me a pink potty which I used for all my three children. Amir said the pink potty was the reason we never had boys.

Early in August, I heard by mail that I had passed. I did not go to the college, which was a common triumphal tradition, but I did hear from one of the beery Australians that Gareth was there with Pat, both wreathed in smiles, he said.

Within the week, I was back in Kampala. At the airport, I saw

Amir in the open receiving area. I could see that he had some apprehension about where my heart was. He must have read between lines in my letters. We went home, and in the first five minutes I was pregnant with my firstborn. I must have timed my return with ovulation, or I could just have risen to the occasion as many primates do. Actions instead of words to assure him that my heart was where it wanted to be.

FOUR

Jinja and Rushna

Jinja

I fully expected to get a medical school-based job. After all, I was amongst the three first registrars trained by the department toward the MRCOG. Gareth Barberton never returned to Uganda, and F. M. Bulwa did not come back till later. So it had to be me. Dr. QS, who had taken over from Coralie, sympathized in the most condescending manner but told me there was no opening. The government-held jobs at Mulago Hospital, Kampala, were also filled. The closest opening was in the Government Hospital in Jinja, fifty miles from Kampala. Also at that time, the owner of a 30-bedded country hospital in Kampala called and tried to persuade me into a private practice, which I was reluctant to embark on. So we decided on Jinja, with Amir and his all-purpose man Husseini commuting the fifty miles to his office in Kampala and then home to Jinja. A hundred miles a day on treacherous roads to accommodate me.

We packed our bags and a few other belongings into the dark blue Peugeot 403 that Amir drove. We also purchased a used Fiat 500, no larger than a medium-sized refrigerator, for my local use in Jinja. I believe it gave about a hundred miles to a gallon of gasoline. And we started our *safari* to Jinja, Amir in the heavily loaded Peugeot and I in my refrigerator. The road was quite level, but if there was even the slightest uphill gradient, I had to stop the car and unload whatever was in the car, and Husseini and Amir carried the unloaded baggage and met me at the top of the hill. One great advantage of this car was that I never had parking problems. If it was improperly parked, two muscular humans could just lift it into place.

So we arrived at our solid spacious government-built house, 145 Jackson Crescent in Jinja. A crescent-shaped driveway led to a stone car-porch opposite the stairs that led to the house. In two large planters arose curving and curling 'money plants,' *philodendron*, curtaining the porch from outside eyes. The heart-shaped leaves of the plant varied from enormous to small, new and wet green. And little yellow-green birds flew in and out of this green curtain. As they came close to the leaves, they would disappear. A closer, quieter look showed many of them entering leaves that had been matched perfectly with a partner and stitched together with some gossamer thread. Tailor birds, we called them—though I cannot locate them in my Birds of East Africa book. I wrote to my in-house poetic bird expert—my nephew Cyrus, my sister Perrin's son. Cyrus knows every birdcall as though it was a voice from his own family and has hawk eyes that, unaided, can discern a speck and a movement from miles away. He reminded me that Kipling in his Jungle Book named the tailor bird *Darzee*.

'The tailor bird neatly sutures together twin leaf blades. It collects spider silk from heaven knows where and uses hair-thin strands to mate the perfectly matched leaf blades into cup-like or pendant-shaped hammocks. This it lines with a silk-cotton bed to house its tiny elliptical shell-brown eggs.' I once picked a fallen leaf-nest, and my prying finger felt the gossamer inside of it. I kept it in my pocket to feel and stroke when the need arose.

The house had an enormous living room and an evil dark kitchen since *memsahibs* did not cook. Our meager belongings occupied a corner of the living room and part of one bedroom. The rest of the house had 'PWD' (Public Works Department) furniture—random chairs and tables that I tried unsuccessfully to create a home with.

That evening I drove over to the maternity wards of the hospital. I was met by a much-relieved medical officer whose Italian background had been in Pathology, but was now in charge of the Obstetrics and Gynecology service. Dr. O's story was that after all these years in Pathology, he wanted to go into a clinical field such as Ob/Gyn and do REAL work and earn REAL money. He had thought a shortcut to gain experience would be to serve in Africa, but never thought he would be the sole person in charge of the Ob/Gyn service. As it was, he had had enough and was to redirect himself into general surgery. He wanted to hand over the service that night, but I declined, saying I'd be in first thing in the morning.

'Before you leave,' he said, 'this patient just came in from the *charo'*—nameless, uncountable and unaccounted villages. She had been in labor several days with the fetal head seen at the perineum during contractions. 'Also no fetal heart.' He led me to a curtained cubicle in the delivery area. I confirmed his findings. Although the fetal head was seen, it was immensely distorted and elongated with most of it felt above the pelvic brim. He and I agreed that the fetal head should be decompressed, thus allowing vaginal delivery. 'Good night and thank you,' said he.

We spent a comfy night in cavernous surroundings. The next morning, Amir left for Kampala, and I went to the hospital early, certain that Dr. O, who was so eager to leave the Ob/Gyn service, would not be there to ease my transition. Not only was that the case, but, as I prepared to round on patients, I found that the patient from the night before was still undelivered. 'We were waiting for you,' I was told.

A dangerous case to start my obstetric life in Jinja. Fetal death was a forgone conclusion, but what if this infected dehydrated woman was lost? A maternal death as my first case was not an easy thought.

I located a perforator, a medieval-looking instrument with a pointed end and cutting edges on the outside of blades.

We positioned the uncomplaining woman. I give her some local anesthesia, and applied conventional obstetric forceps—correctness of application was irrelevant in this long-dead fetus—to steady the head. An assistant held the handles of the forceps as I directed the perforator to the fetal skull, protecting maternal tissues with my

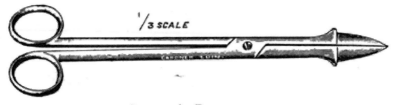

SMELLIE'S PERFORATOR.

left hand. A sharp movement, and I entered the fetal cranium with the perforator. I opened the blades, allowing the cutting edges to tear an opening in the skull. I then rotated the instrument through a right angle and repeated the process.

'A cruciate opening does the job best,' rang in my ears from some previous teacher.

Then the liquefied brain started falling out. I helped the process. Soon, enough material had escaped to allow the head to collapse and descend. Tissue forceps with fierce grasping teeth were applied to the opening in the skull, and with gentle traction on the obstetric forceps, the head was delivered. The poor relieved body just fell into waiting arms. No one in the room thought upon this heinous procedure. Just relief all around because it was over.

I had to move on. A ward full of patients, and a clinic waiting. Cases to book for the next day's surgery.

It is difficult to imagine that I was pregnant with my most squeamish of daughters, Rushna, when I performed this procedure. Conveniently blunted sensitivity helped me to disassociate.

Jinja: Nalin and Kamalaben

Nalin Choksi, a year junior to us in medical school, lived and practiced in Jinja. Amir and he had a special bond because, at one time as medical students, they were both in love with the same nurse, Amir for a short time and Nalin for longer. When the nurse became an airline stewardess, Nalin would spend his off-time at airports watching the planes come in the random hope that she would be on one of them.

A bachelor, he lived with his formidable mother Kamalaben, a prototype of the tough East African Asian woman. She was small dark round and firm. She wore starched white saris, in *sidha* style, the old-fashioned way loosely over the right shoulder, rather than the modern figure revealing style. A bunch of keys always rattled at her waist, and she kept account of each lentil and grain of rice. She ran this spotless vegetarian—it was interesting to see even the dog eat rice and *dal* (spicy yellow lentils) household with her two sons, one daughter-in-law and a bevy of girl grandchildren.

The amazing thing about Kamalaben was that after her husband's death, she trained as a midwife and supported her large family while they were young and in school. She was the midwife for the Jinja Asian women who preferred home delivery. While most Asian women of her time never worked outside the home, she continued this active life, often coming home in the mornings sleepless and tired, but ready for another day of strict household management. She was respected and adored by her sons and by me, but probably only respected by her daughter-in-law.

Nalin would often come to 145 Jackson Crescent for dinner, and the three of us had long companiable evenings. One of our favorite evening pastimes was to sit by Lake Victoria and watch the daily evening thunder and lightning shows, more impressive than any *son-et-lumière* I have ever seen. Disturbed by the lightning, we would hear snorts, and out would lumber families of hippopotami, which we watched secretly from the bushes.

When I was about eight weeks pregnant and pitifully nauseous, I had some spotting. Nervous about my previous pregnancy loss, I took to bed for a few days. The help we had would kindly put a gardenia from the garden in a small vase near my bed, and to this day the smell of gardenias makes me nauseous. Since Amir was away during the day, Nalin dropped by at lunchtime to check on me and bring some of Kamalaben's vegetarian specials.

My spotting soon stopped and I was back to work. I made the most of Amir's indulgence and asked him to bring fanciful things from Kampala. But when I saw them in the evening, the passion for them was gone. Once, he often reminded me, I asked for chocolate-covered ginger, and then added, 'And don't expect me to eat them.' I ate atrociously in the first trimester. All I recall eating greedily in the first three months was raw mango with masses of salt and fiery hot chilli powder, which Rushna, the fetus I was then harboring, adores to this day.

Amir and I had a rudimentary knowledge of chess, taught to us by his sister Laila and her future husband, Aneel. We started playing every evening, and my recollection is that he never won till much later, when Rushna was born. After that, my distraction totally precluded winning. Who says motherhood can't dumb you down?

Jinja: Independence Day — The day her uterus ruptured

Uganda was to be declared an independent nation on October 9, 1962. As appropriate, all the makings of a democracy started to emerge. Apollo Milton Obote was the Chairman of the Uganda Peoples Congress (UPC) with its widest base outside the Kampala area. The opposition Democratic Party (DP), with Benedicto Kiwanuka as chairman, represented the Catholic Baganda and the Asians. As mentioned earlier, the traditional King of Buganda, the Kabaka, an Anglican, was a power amongst the Baganda people, a highly educated, sophisticated and powerful group. To legitimize them, the Kabaka and followers formed a third party, the Kabaka Yekka (KY). Amir always said that 'yekka' was a mystical word, difficult to translate, but meaning, more or less, the Kabaka one and alone. Elections were planned prior to Independence to give order to this fledgling democracy. Infighting in the UPC caused Obote, chairman of the UPC, and Jolly Joe Kiwanuka, the president of the UPC, to mutually fire each other, but Obote prevailed and became the undisputed power in the UPC. The Kabaka boycotted the elections and all the seats in Buganda went by default to Benedicto Kiwanuka and the DP. Thus, Bendicto Kiwanuka became the first elected Prime Minister of not yet independent Uganda with Obote as the leader of the opposition.

To settle their differences, the warring factions were invited to Lancaster House, a conference mediated by Iain Macleod, the Colonial Secretary. It was clear that no progress could be made unless the Kabaka was placated. In a stroke of genius, Obote proposed that the Kabaka be made president of Uganda and the UPC form an alliance with the KY party, with a promise from KY not to independently contest the election, which would split the vote. With this arrangement, the 1962 elections were held, and Obote's UPC party with its KY coalition, riding on the Baganda votes, easily defeated DP's Bendicto Kiwanuka. In addition to the Kabaka being President, the KY party was rewarded with five ministerial positions, including the powerful Ministry of Finance.

Whatever. There was general euphoria at all this being settled, ruling one's own house. And there was the innocent promise of a democratic multiracial society, with blacks and Asians living

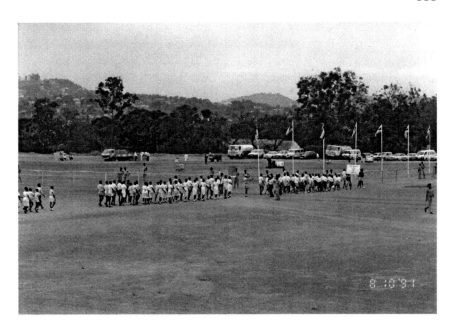

together and the British gracefully receding. While many Asians were considering, Amir and I changed our citizenship from British to Ugandan as soon as we could.

October 9th, 1962. As always, night fell like a curtain in this country with no twilight. We drove to Kampala from Jinja, and as we approached the city, scores of people in their creative brightnesses joined the crowds at the Lugogo parade grounds. Thirty years later, we happened on Kampala on another October 9th. It was astounding to see the same friendly crowds, the same singing schoolchildren.

Years of killings and HIV had not robbed this day of its magic. We are resilient beyond all limits.

As midnight approached, two men walked to the dais, where the Union Jack and the Crested Crane fluttered. The one, white tall upper class, being a good old boy till the end, aquiline nose— who was it? Prince Philip? A prototype, anyway. Resplendent in a whiter-than-gleaming white naval uniform with dazzling epaulets and medallions. And next to him, in business suit, a civilian, *mwana inchi*—a man of the people, that black profile, the nose the very antithesis of the other. I felt for that lonely man accepting the country. We would see to him. We would not make his a lonely task. Midnight and God Save the Queen. And then up rose the young Crane in gold and black. The Ugandan national anthem in English sounded tinny and naïve. I am always stirred by national anthems in languages I do not understand. It's the same as loving opera in Italian but finding it embarrassingly trite in English.

'Oh Uganda! May God uphold thee
We lay our future in thy hand
United, free
For liberty
Together we'll always stand.' etc.

The unmelodic wail gave me some misgivings. Put it aside. The glory was that the British had once more left. Enjoy.

It was about one in the morning when we drove the fifty miles back to Jinja. We swerved and swayed to the tune of *waragi*-filled revelers on the red dirt siding by the road. My feelings were of tolerance and euphoria from the scenes of a few moments ago. The strutting crested crane framed in bright colors.

When we arrived back at our Jinja home, a hospital messenger lay asleep on our doorstep with the call book open on his torso. The message read:

"Patient brought in by taxi. Nine months pregnant, no antenatal care. In labor for five days. Local remedies tried. Still undelivered. BP 80/?, Pulse 140/min, temp 101 degrees F, Abdomen tense and tender. No fetal heart heard.

Vaginal examination—Fully dilated with fetal shoulder and arm prolapsed into the vagina.

Antibiotics, fluids started, blood being matched. Operating theatre ready. Awaiting MD."

While I was exulting on the British departure, this woman was laboring, close to death, with a transversely lying fetus. Who was on call? No matter. The message indicated the best we could offer had been done. On the short drive to the hospital I tried to figure out the crucial question. Had the uterus ruptured? If it had not, then vaginal delivery after embryotomy—dismembering the fetus—was her best chance. If it had ruptured this procedure would extend the injury in the uterus and further threaten this fragile life.

At the hospital the stalwart writer of the note had made the judgment that the uterus was ruptured. The patient was already on the operating room table. A cursory examination, and I quickly agreed.

There were two medical assistants to manage the patient with me. One was the anesthetist and the other the operating room technologist. I knew them both as cool and efficient men who had helped through several emergencies.

The anesthetist spoke quietly and sweetly to the woman as he started general anesthesia. The tech and I scrubbed. He was unusually quiet, and I interpreted this as anger at my late arrival. The patient was intubated and maintained on a mixture of ether and air.

I started as I was taught by Professor Coralie, who was the world's authority on ruptured uterus. Maximum vertical incision. A long-dead fetus was extruded into the peritoneal cavity—no sentimentality allowed—deliver and forget it. Into a bucket it went. The placenta was floating free—get rid of it. Bring the uterus into the incision, and pause to define the edges of the tear. Relief—the urinary bladder was intact. The tear had savaged the uterus, and a hysterectomy would have been best. But the pressures of society favored a woman who menstruated, even if infertile. So I started the lesser procedure of repair of the uterine rupture and tubal ligation. She could not be allowed to get pregnant again as the scar would heal poorly and inevitably rupture with another pregnancy.

I became aware of my assistant's swaying and giggling and general lack of reaction to our dire problem. 'Retractor,' I said. 'Okay,' he said in an exaggerated way. No retractor. My paranoia—was he really saying, 'This is the 10th of October 1962, and I don't have to take anything from you'? I nervously looked up at the anesthetist. He silently lifted his thumb up to his mouth and closed his eyes, indicating 'drunk.' Drunk! I plodded on, reaching for instruments myself. The tray was lacking most of what I needed. The hot-water sterilizer was immediately outside the operating room. Flushed with frustration, I started to make trips to get what I needed. This was a doomed patient. On my third trip to the sterilizer my eyes fell on a telephone. I picked it up in my bloody gloved hands, scrub be damned. Operator, operator—an answer! I called Amir from his slumber to come help. He dashed over in my Fiat 500.

Doctor though he was, large quantities of blood terrified him. He also had no clue when it came to the names of surgical instruments. So I called for instruments by description. The long-handled things with the 'O's at the end, the short-handled things with teeth. He was speedy, and his errors were made up for by speed. My giggling friend stayed put retracting and was fine as long as I did not ask him to move.

Using thick chromic catgut, I sutured the ragged tear in the uterus. I picked up the poor Fallopian tubes that were not to function as conduits any longer. I washed out the abdomen with gallons of saline and closed hurriedly, all in one layer.

The dear anesthetist told me to go home. He would manage. My husband was on the verge of something close to total collapse. I accepted the offer, and we fell into a deep sleep as soon as we got home to our bed.

The next day, independence euphoria was already a bit ragged. I walked into the office of the chief medical officer to complain. He smiled and said that I had to understand that Independence Day was once in a lifetime. His look plainly told me that I, of a different race, was not expected to participate or understand. Not black enough and never white enough.

To prove his point and prove that I was stressing without reason, the patient gradually recovered with no lasting problems and soon waved goodbye.

Jinja: Tejani reunion

Happiness. I had the partner I needed, a daughter was on her way, I was not nauseous but ravenous, I had a job where I actually saved lives, I lived in a big rambling house, the raucous Tejanis were fifty miles away and yet right there when there was fun to be had. And a five-minute trip took me to the source of the Nile and bathing hippos. I lived in an independent country with an elected government and aspirations of multiracial harmony.

Christmas 1962 brought the whole Tejani clan to Jinja for unabated revelry. Haruna was the name of our house help. If there was a lull in the proceedings, the code cry would be 'Haruna! *Lete* cider!' and the Bulmer's cider and much else flowed. I seemed to have an internal alert when I was pregnant that would cause nausea with the slightest drop of alcohol—much before the knowledge of the toxic effects of alcohol on pregnancy. I could use it as a pregnancy test, it was so reliable.

Nalin was a constant visitor during this time. One evening, during the Tejani revelries, he brought a pediatrician friend, AV, whom he consulted on complicated pediatric cases. To illustrate the complex lives we led, AV started talking about his club.

'Club?' I asked. 'Isn't that a restricted whites-only affair?'

'Yes,' he said, without the faintest embarrassment.

Here he was in our home and yet he did not get the grossness of it. I indulged in one of my worst habits, stirring up things and then walking away from confrontation. I do not think Amir even noticed at first. He had grown up in this country and exclusive clubs were just there to be accepted. So I started in on the man who proceded to use arguments such as 'Anyone was welcome to start a club and exclude others.' He invited me to start one since I seemed to pine to belong to one and then, he said, I could have the pleasure of excluding him. I was dumbfounded, but Amir took on the cause in loud and definitely obnoxious terms, as only he could. In the end, AV spluttered to me, 'Your husband is a rabble rouser,' and left.

The process of bias and prejudice would be interesting if it were not the deadliest sin.

1963 — Jinja: Abdominal pregnancy

Staff Nurse Irene Kigonde was one of those starched smiling shining people, who, in even terms and tone, placated patients and nurses and doctors. She would look out for me to make our rounds, and whatever the time, she would be there to help carry out our plans. And she was always there. Never 'called in sick' and appeared never to take vacation. Just raise your head when you needed her, and she would materialize, anticipating what had to be done.

Irene once walked onto the ward with a patient from the clinic, saying she wanted me to examine her. All was not well, she said. The patient claimed that she was way past her due date. She based this conviction on unconfirmable events. The purchase of a chicken, the second pounding of the cassava. Not even a vague date for her last menstrual period. In a life of subsistence, a menstrual period is of little import. She had taken the traditional medicine, *dagara kiganda*, to bring on labor with no results. Our hospital was her last resort. She felt the baby move, but feared its death if the pregnancy continued.

Any probing into her dates offended her. She had told Irene that the village women teased her about being closer to an elephant (gestational age one year) than a human. I asked Irene: She may be past her due date, what's so unusual? Irene said, 'Feel her abdomen.' It is embarrassing how one has to be reminded of such basics.

After Irene's admonition I did indeed feel her abdomen. There was a smooth mass on the right. Fibroid, I thought. A fetus was vaguely felt on the left. The bugle fetoscope elicited a fetal heartbeat. A wildly unusual pelvic examination showed the cervix tucked way up under the pubic bones and continuous with the mass on the right. There was a round firm structure behind the cervix that could only be a fetal head. The mass on the right was the empty uterus, and the fetus lay free in the abdomen on the left. An abdominal pregnancy! A long-ago embryo implanted in a tube and then grown or ruptured into the abdomen, and instead of the usually catastrophic ruptured ectopic pregnancy, continued to grow undisturbed with

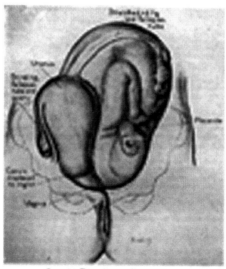

the placenta doing a gallant job amongst organs not designed to feed it. I looked incredulously at Irene. Some people are gifted with clinical brilliance quite apart from book-learnt knowledge. Without her astuteness I can imagine this patient suffering through days of unsuccessful attempts at induction of labor.

We conveyed our suspicions to the patient, who took a commonsense approach. 'Just do your job and get me over this ridiculous pregnancy.'

Armed with several units of blood, I explored her abdomen. Like a bride veiled in a glistening sheet of fat-speckled omentum this fetus lay, its head burrowed deep in the pelvis between the urinary bladder in front and the rectum behind, with the uterus banished to the right. The baby lay in a sac that had been fortified with inflammatory secretions, ingenuously passing for amniotic fluid.

Wake up, baby, rid yourself of endorphins and arrive. A gentle dissection freed the head, and the body slithered into waiting arms. The cord was clamped and the baby was lusty—almost relieved.

Where lay the placenta? This was the moment for which blood was in readiness. The thin irregularly shaped placenta had spread itself over the outside of the uterus, the shiny layer of peritoneum lining the abdomen and the omentum. To leave it in and risk infection or to peel it off and risk hemorrhage was the dilemma. A main vascular channel appeared to supply it. After clamping this, we slowly and gingerly peeled off this unique placenta. We were soon done and ready to close.

Contemplate the baby. A few pressure effects of lying in its cozy but immobile position. Memories of continuous pressure from mother's organs left an asymmetric jaw and ears that did not quite match. Nothing that time would not smooth away.

The human condition was manufactured with fetal isolation in mind. Isolated undisturbed and alone. Even a partner twin causes crowding. How did this one adapt to gurgling gut, moving and swishing around, a restless urinary bladder that filled and emptied, filled and emptied. An ornamental omental blanket with fetal feet warmed in mother's soft liver. An umbilical cord coiling and swirling free.

The patient was told of Irene's role in the diagnosis. She

rewarded us and burdened the baby by calling her Irene Tejani Nsubuga.

Jinja: A maternal death

My last menstrual period was on Indian Independence day, August 15th, making me due on May 22nd. I had a yen to show my father my pregnant persona, so I decided to quit working in the end of April to visit him before I had the baby.

I was particularly happy that I had steered through the complicated busy Jinja months without a death on either the obstetric or gynecologic service. And then it happened. That desperate obstetric hemorrhage.

Over decades of practice, across time and continents, the red scenes of obstetric hemorrhage remain in the memory—written in indelible letters. The incredible pregnant uterus clamps down at the moment of delivery and applies a myriad tourniquets around blood vessels that have generously fed the fetus till moments before.

During the course of a pregnancy, the blood supply to the uterus has increased from negligible to enormous. It is enough to quickly exsanguinate, even bleed to death, if the natural tourniquets do not clamp down. Clotting magic then helps until the uterus returns to its quiescent stance. The clotting process may also be disrupted, and bleeding behind the placenta may 'use up' the coagulative proteins. Occasionally a message of amniotic fluid is delivered into the mother's circulation through a fault line in the amniotic membranes. Amniotic fluid has powerful anticoagulant properties and unmatchable hemorrhage results.

She came in by taxi from a nearby village hospital. She was pale, a gray opaque color, and sweaty, a pulse scarcely felt and a blood pressure not forceful enough to supply her vital organs. Her uterus was tense and exquisitely tender. No fetus could be felt because of the tenseness of the uterus, and no fetal heartbeat could be heard.

Excessive bleeding from all puncture sites where blood samples had been taken and intra-venous infusions started heralded the worst. Her placenta had separated prematurely, and her blood had been leached of all its coagulative factors and had lost the ability to clot. A tube of her blood taped to the wall refused to clot.

She was almost too fragile to be touched. We poured in un-crossmatched universal donor blood while further units of blood were being matched.

There was a flicker of response. A pelvic examination showed that her cervix was fully dilated and the long-dead fetus was making its ultimate journey. She soon delivered with the completely separated placenta delivered with the innocent. And the bleeding! Not the reassuring syrupy stuff but a watered-down pinkish substitute. Watery unclotted blood poured from her uterus and seeping from all the injection sites. And she had poison pink urine. No time to mop, no time to clean. A red tide.

She was too sick for surgery, and we tried to pack her uterus to tamponade the bleeding. But the packing was soaked as it was being introduced and practically washed out in the ferocity of the hemorrhage.

It was impossible to stand and watch. A swift hysterectomy seemed a last desperate chance.

There was bleeding from everywhere as I entered the abdomen. A few clamps and the womb was detached from its stays.

Could it be possible? The bleeding appeared to have stopped. I looked up at the anesthestist. 'I'm trying, I'm trying,' his eyes told me. He poured in fluids, blood, plasma. We were losing her. No pressure, no bleeding. Suddenly, surgery was simplified. Visibility was perfect. She had left.

In these parts, news of dire events travel on invisible lines. I heard wails and an ululatory lament reserved for catastrophe. Almost never had I been the first to communicate bad news. They already knew.

I left the operating room to look. The woman was the mother of six children. But through the moans, I saw the villagers close ranks. She did not have six children—they had six children. They would be cared for in poverty's generous way.

Leaving Jinja

This last event left me sad and unhappy. For reasons that seem obvious but hard to explain, managing a maternal death by a very pregnant obstetrician has to be an unhealthy experience. I wanted to leave and yet I wanted to stay and leave on a happier note. My time in Jinja, otherwise happy, had started with the neglected patient where I had to decompress the fetal head for delivery and ended with this death. That's it.

Dr. O and his American wife who spent all her time reading magazines at the hotel pool invited us for a goodbye meal. There were no other guests, and I had been previously told that we were the only people still friendly with him, mainly because he did not do any obstetrics. He once asked to scrub with me on a myomectomy, removal of fibroids from a fibroid-studded uterus. His wild and uncontrolled movements made me so nervous that I took over. He later admonished me for not being able to teach surgery. And I was glad never to see him again over a surgical table. Lack of contact maintained our friendship.

The meal was a several-course Italian affair with antipasto, pasta, meat and then a dessert and espresso. At the end of this, the poor man waiting at the table plonked down a green salad in front of each of us. Mrs. O had told him to serve it after the main course and since he had forgotten ('It's all mixed up in the end'), he brought it after coffee. At first I thought this may be an Italian thing. But then I saw Mrs. O turn color and let out a scream of abuse the likes of which I never want to see or hear again. 'It all gets mixed up in the end' did not work.

Goodbye, Irene, star of the staff nurses, and then we left.

A last time with my father

Amir drove me to Nairobi for a few days together, and we took our usual drive of enchantment through the game park before I boarded the Air India plane to Bombay, Pune and Mahableshwar. Pune (previously Poona of P.G. Wodehouse Poona colonel fame), 120 miles from Bombay over the Western Ghats, the palisade that edges the western margin of the mainland, was a cool escape from the sultry heat of Bombay. My father's brother Eruch, a slight shadow of a man who shook your hand like the touch of a moth, lived in Pune with his robust and tough wife Soona and their four children. Soona Aunty kept a buffalo tied up in the backyard whom she personally milked. Buffalo milk has a huge fat content (12%

versus a cow's 4%). From this, she would make her own butter and ghee. She also had a chicken coop with large birds strutting about with names like Rhode Island Red, Black Minorca and White Leghorn. Every morning she would collect these enormous eggs for our breakfast.

One morning I heard the usual clucking indicating eggs were being laid. But one bird's insistent clucking caught Soona Aunty's attention. She said in Gujerati that she heard trouble. I followed her out to the insistent clucking from a great White Leghorn who was obviously distressed. Without any preliminaries Soona Aunty put her hand into the bird's vagina. She explained to me that the egg was lying across instead of pointed end down. A transverse lie, in obstetric terms. She did a quick internal version to convert it to the correct position, and out plopped a warm egg for our breakfast.

Soona Aunty's idea of scrambled eggs was several fresh large eggs, with masses of ghee and cream churned from her own buffalo. A few bites of this was enough to clog the arteries forever.

While I was there, Soona and Eruch's children put on a concert to celebrate returning the money they had borrowed from my father decades ago for the purchase of the rambling house they lived in. Their daughter Mehru, fair and freckled with long curly brown hair, had the loveliest of soprano voices and sang old English and French ditties and an Italian aria or two with her sister and two brothers helping as chorus. Then the check was presented with a flourish and a long and loving letter. My father, never expecting the money back, looked so quiet and peaceful. Much happier here than in the lonely life he led in Bombay.

Matriarchal Soona could not and would not let her children leave to better their lives. Mehru of the golden voice had a chance to study at the conservatory in Paris and Soona would not hear of it. One of her sons applied to medical school and got a spot in a city a few hours from Pune. Once again she could not allow this. My uncle had a law degree, but lacked the confidence to practice. He lived his whole life as an underpaid, overworked Crachitt-like clerk and certainly had no say in his children's future. And the children accepted and loved their mother no matter what. Till today, long after her death.

There is a traditional Parsi ceremony called 'kisi koti' (literally 'hugs and kisses') performed at all happy occasions, birthdays, weddings and welcoming back family, specially if pregnant. So in Bombay at my grandmother's house, in Pune at my Aunt's place and in Mahableshwar at my niece's, before I crossed the threshold that was decorated with chalk stencils in 'lucky' shapes of fish and stars, a garland of roses and tuberoses was put around my neck, a red dot planted on my forehead, a piece of rock sugar put in my mouth with a sip of milk, a coconut and perfect heart-shaped betel nut leaves placed in my hands. Rose-water was sprinkled and rice was generously scattered over me and prolonged kisses and hugs (thus the *kisi koti*) given. Everyone in the welcoming group did this separately, so the whole thing could be fairly prolonged. The full original ceremony also involved breaking an egg at the threshold, but in the interest of preventing an eggy mess, this part was scratched. In an abbreviated way I have done this for my children and their children to everyone's delight. People ask me the significance, and I come up with many nonsense things, mainly wishes for fertility which obviously did not apply to very pregnant me.

It was time to leave. I wanted to roam no more but to stay still with Amir. So goodbye to all in India. And specially a last goodbye to my father, who never saw any of my children.

I arrived in Nairobi where Amir had driven down with all his sibs and Husseni to meet me. They had spent a few days at the Serengeti Game Park in Tanzania before coming to meet my plane. At the airport I saw Amir in his car, but he would not do his usual bounding down to meet me. I walked over to the car and saw that he was shirtless and had on a tiny pair of rumpled striped cotton shorts held up by a tatty drawstring. 'I have no pants,' he said, explaining why he would not get out of the car. Feeling hot, he had taken them off, and instead of guarding them, he left them in a second car, which Husseni had allowed sister Sultan to drive. She had overturned it about five miles from the airport. No one was hurt, and they gleefully took pictures of the car before they got help to right it. They soon arrived, Amir retrieved his pants, and we drove back to Kampala.

Rushna

While I had been away, Amir had rented a semi-detached house on Lower Kololo Terrace on Baskerville Avenue. A small garden led up to a polished red-floored patio which entered into a long living and dining room. A doorway led to two bedrooms and a dismal kitchen at the far end. Almost unbelievably when we entered, I heard the Beatles complaining of A Hard Day's Night. Come evening, the battling started, only now there was a ten-year-old son participating in the arguments. I had never noticed the son at our previous apartment. As the night progressed and his parents suddenly became quiet, he switched on the Beatles and listened and sang in peace. We and the Scottish couple were back together, side by side.

Two weeks after my due date, on the 2nd of June 1963, a Sunday night, I started labor. I was astounded, shocked, unbelieving at what labor felt like. In my wildest dreams I never expected it to be so painful. I had always thought I was one of those 'can do anything' types, but this was close to defeating me. Recently a male medical student told me his impressions of the first delivery he had seen. He was shocked and said he thought the whole thing very badly designed. Indeed.

Even worse, when I arrived at Mulago Hospital and was examined by a midwife, my cervix had not even started dilating.

The interminable night ended and Daphne Kayton arrived in the morning to tell me my cervix was effacing, but not dilating. All morning, Daphne, Amir and I walked up and down the wide open, airy corridors of the hospital. And then came lunchtime. My obstetrician and my husband went out to lunch, leaving me to myself—unbelievable. Twenty-nine years later, Rushna, my first born, had just had her second baby, and her husband Kevin and I went out to lunch while she scowled and smoldered at the unfairness of it.

Amir came back from lunch somewhat shame-faced with a fruit tart for me. No 'fluids only' in labor in those days, and I consumed it quickly. As another night fell (who said, 'Never let the sun set twice on a laboring woman'?) my contractions started doing some real work, and my cervix finally gave up and started dilating. In

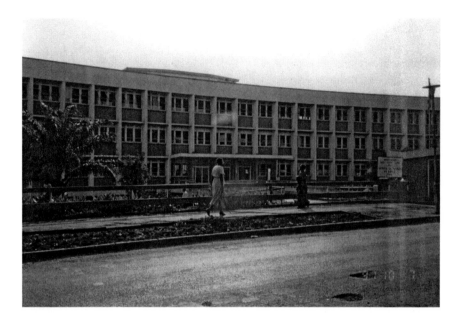

the early hours of June 4th morning, I received my one and only sedation—25mgs of Pethidine (Demarol). Twenty-five mgs and yet this made me sleep soundly between contractions. I woke up to one contraction and saw Amir reading the comic strip in a newspaper. I still flush at the rage I felt and expressed. On reflection it wasn't the darned comic strip. Just the enormity of this deep dark pain. He was shocked at me and the comic strip disappeared, and I sank into sleep. And then that uncontrollable urge to push. I have never been able to fathom women who will not push at full dilatation. There was no controlling me. I was taken to the delivery room and moved onto the table where I was to have all three of my babies. No lithotomy position for me. Just drew my legs up when I felt the urge.

Daphne suggested I use the trilene mask. The idea was to inhale trilene gas when the contraction started so that the peak of pain is not felt when you temporarily reach unconsciousness and the mask falls away. Amir in his eagerness to help put the mask on me upside down (nose end toward my chin), obstructing my breathing and thus my decision not to use that evil-sounding thing. An acme of pain and the head and then that unforgettable slither against the

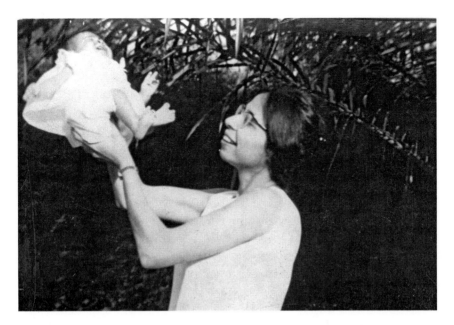

inner part of my thigh. I have rolled the memory of three slithers into one glorious one. The tears could not be held back. Rushna, my first born. The eighteenth day of the Parsi calendar is Rashne. Rushne Rast—the Parsi angel of Justice.

'Walking on air,' said Amir, 'Walking on air.' And he never came down.

I, however, quickly came down from airy heights as my large medio-lateral episiotomy was being put together, preventing me from sitting normally for a month. I vowed never to inflict a medio-lateral on any but my worst enemies. And since my worst enemies never came to me for delivery, I never inflicted this medieval cut on anyone. I took a good sentimental look at my placenta and thanked it for its stalwart performance.

My perfect little Rushna was born with a loose incisor tooth that had to be lifted off by a dentist before I could settle into six months of breast feeding. I was at home for a month, during which time Rushna cried continuously, particularly at night. I later discovered it might have been the caffeine in the twenty cups of tea I drank each day. Rushna can still make night into day partying, a leftover from my caffeine-soaked mothering. I buried her umbilical cord stump under a pink hibiscus bush in the front yard. I recall incessant flowering ever since.

Naipaul and us

Some months after Rushna was born, my obstetrician and friend Daphne Kayton gave me V. S. Naipaul's 'An Area of Darkness.' Amir and I took opposite sides on this book and every other book he wrote after that. Naipaul was a thread through our lives that never failed to cause us to spend time and more time trying to untangle our mixed and complicated feelings about him. We agreed on his mastery of the language—and disagreed about all else. To me it seemed that after brief travels in India and later East Africa, Iran, Indonesia and Pakistan, he made fast destructive judgments on their mired and hopeless condition permanently warped by colonial masters, but defective even without. Contempt. He held all he met in contempt. How can a writer of human behaviour become great without empathy? And yet, I confess, he did show empathy, softest humor and what was it—a feeling for 'my people,' a sentiment that he would no doubt scorn—in his earlier Trinidad books, and in the letters to his father and treatment of his brother Shiva. I was introduced to Shiva's writing in a cottage in Tobago. The small library contained 'The Divi Divi Trees.' Shiva wrote with the usual qualities of heart and soul. Easy to follow, easy to like. But ordinary.

Why did we constantly stress about Naipaul? There was an odd pride in this grandson of Indian immigrants—worse, indentured workers, a parallel with Amir. Perhaps it was this that made him a compelling presence in our lives and those of Amir's brothers and sisters. The physically closest we had ever been was while Naipaul was writer-in-residence at Makerere University in Kampala. I never set eyes on him, but Bahadur, who taught at Makerere, gave the opinion I heard again and again over the years, that he was superior, intolerant, and contemptuous—all the opposite qualities one expects of someone who makes his living as an observer of humans. Bahadur, who is also endowed with a sizeable ego, was probably completely ignored by this acerb who refused to treat other people of similar color as brothers. Asians in Uganda generally felt this compelling closeness and could not tolerate rebuffs from other Asians.

I read later that Naipaul had taught at Wesleyan College in Middletown, Connecticut, in the 80's. He was remembered as an unpleasant terror and a most unpedogogic presence—a man who regarded the constant sea of young people around him as contaminating.

Paul Theroux started off as Naipaul's self-appointed protégé when they first met at Makerere University in Kampala, but was impelled to write a peevish account of their relationship after he fell out of favor. Once over tea at the Charing Cross Hotel, they saw a 'heavily pregnant woman.' Theroux quoted Naipaul, 'To me, one of the ugliest sights on earth is a pregnant woman.' To me, one of the sweetest sights on earth is the pregnant woman. She softens in my eyes with the first positive pregnancy test and rapidly diminishes after the birth of the baby. I start losing interest even before the placenta is out—a dangerous attitude for an obstetrician. But another reason to deeply dislike Naipaul.

There was derision, providing some relief, since it was a common feeling between Amir and me, when Naipaul accepted knighthood. From then on, we would mock him—Sir Vidya. Not even the Nobel retrieved him in our eyes.

Kennedy African style

November 22 1963. I heard the ululations long before I knew. Long low echoing pangs of grief. They came from somewhere in the valley below. A woman started and before she tailed off another took it on. Then a deeper male voice. Death cries. A death in the little settlement in the valley. Who could it be that affected the whole village? A child that had become a collective joint family child? An elder who was head of the whole village? Surely someone who touched many lives. The wails, filled with staccato grief, now came from a different end of the valley, and soon we were surrounded by a curtain of voices, all expressing loss.

This was not a 'daily' death. It had to be something else. As people of Indian origin in a newly independent African country, even while proclaiming our allegiance we were nervous. The party in power, the UPC, with Obote at the helm, seemed reasonable and even tolerated some mild opposition. Was some juggling occurring at the top?

We switched on to Radio Uganda. Mournful music and then a choking voice in English with African intonation could hardly finish his sentences. Kennedy was dead. John Kennedy was dead. Shot in the head in that gun-infested country. 'Our Kennedy was dead,' he said.

My first child was born in June of the year he died. He died a day after my birthday. He died on the day when as young lovers, years before, we had decided to marry. Kennedy and us—we were connected.

I bundled up my five-month-old, and we accompanied Amir to the clinic he ran in the *charo*—a village about ten miles from Kampala. Holding the baby, I walked into the village while he was busy with patients.

There was an old woman with a few vegetables spread out on a striped cloth on the dirt by the roadside. Kneeling next to her was a younger woman. The older woman was clutching a framed picture of smiling Kennedy with shining white teeth. She was talking, explaining to the younger woman. A conversation sprinkled with '*Mukhade, mukhade*' 'Alas, alas.'

These were poor folk, not political. Why did they care so much? America had seeped into the African countryside. When a patient was being discharged from hospital and enquired what she could drink, she would ask, Water? Milk? Pepsi?

That smiling privileged face in the hands of an old woman on no more than subsistence, no envy, but just a strange kind of awe… and love. Could he ever have thought that his image had spread deep into rural Africa, a continent he must rarely have thought about?

In the days that followed, many images—that tragic intensely beautiful Jackie with blood-stained pink suit, bewildered Lyndon Johnson, Oswald dying before our eyes, Ruby from out of nowhere perpetrating the deed. All those commissions that investigated useless theories.

The old vegetable seller's wrinkled mahogany face, smiling photograph in hand, told a strange story— a story of that sub-sect of the privileged who have liberal hearts that appeal to every level.

Years later, in 1972, I stood at his eternal flame at Arlington National Cemetery with Amir, nine-year-old Rushna, six-year-old Cena and four-year-old Sharyn. By this time, Robert lay under a simple white cross near him. Enough.

1964: Private practice

Breast-feeding was going fine and I stopped consuming masses of tea. As a result the poor child established a restful sleep-wake pattern. I reapplied for a government job at Mulago Hospital and was appointed as a 'special grade medical officer' in the Department of Obstetrics and Gynecology. I remember this time as torn and disorganized. It was my first experience of juggling child-care with a round-the-clock obstetrics existence. Much later, long years of the regimen made me better at it, but this first time I wanted to be at home with the baby when at work and wanted to be at work when Rushna tried my patience at home.

A few months of this and I was told that I was to be posted back to Jinja. Another obstetrician, Dr. Shirish Clerk, was to replace me. His great asset was his wife Rashmi, who was an accomplished anesthesiologist which the hospital badly needed. I felt no anger at this because, for the first time, I was not enjoying my job and also because Shirish and Rashmi were old friends some years senior to us from our medical school. Years later, Shirish happened to be passing by when I was fully dilated, and came in and delivered my baby Sharyn. My obstetrician was nowhere to be found. And then a few years after this, after we had already left for the U.S., we heard that Shirish's brother Anil Clerk, a lawyer and friend of Milton Obote, was taken from his home by Idi Amin's special forces, never to be seen again. Anil's wife was in the coastal Kenyan city of Mombasa visiting her parents, having just delivered their first child. After a painful but fruitless search, she emigrated to Toronto and made a life for herself as a pathologist. The son, who never really saw his father, recently graduated from medical school and is on his way to becoming an orthopedic surgeon in the U.S.

We just could not accept going back to Jinja. I guess there must have been some anger at being brushed off again. So, though I was loath to give up a teaching environment, I embarked on a private practice.

Amir knew my misgivings and said he would make it good for me. And he did. We rented three large rooms on the second floor of the pink stone Bank of Baroda building on Kampala Road, the main road that ran through town. The first room was a spacious waiting room with basket chairs and a receptionist. The second was a wood-lined consultation room with a giant rosewood desk, and the third was an examination room with an examination table, a stool and a magnificent light. A corner of this room was a mini-laboratory where I could perform urinanalysis, check hemoglobins and hematocrits with a manual hemoglobinometer. I also had a binocular microscope which I earnestly used for urine sediments, trichomonas and post-coital tests.

For deliveries and gynecologic surgery I used a small thirty-bed country hospital called Nile Nursing Home, run by a Dr. Singh. The surgeon who used this facility was Dr. Manubhai Patel, who practiced one floor above me in the bank building.

The years in private practice, 1964-1970, were the only time I felt the desperate professional isolation that comes with doctoring without company, witness, colleagues, students or teachers. I faithfully read the 'Journal of Obstetrics and Gynaecology of the British Empire'! As the empire dwindled, the name changed to the less ostentatious 'Journal of Obstetrics and Gynaecology of the British Commonwealth.' I believe it is now just plain 'British Journal of Obstetrics and Gynaecology'or BJOG. I published my 'book' commentary of complications following abdominal gynecologic surgery in the 'East African Medical Journal.' The disease of yearning to see my name and work in print started then and never abated.

In my private practice isolation, I put together poorly written pointless observations on cervical incompetence (my only strength was that Dr. V. N. Shirodkar, the 'inventor' of this procedure, was once my teacher) and some case reports. All were rejected by the British Empire.

Sugar daughter

My practice picked up but was humdrum and never overwhelming. I would leave the scarcely year-old Rushna at home with an ayah at about nine in the morning, then drive to the Nile Nursing Home to round on delivered patients, who stayed in for five days, and on recently operated patients. I charged all of 350 shillings ($11) for a delivery and 800 shillings (about $26) for a hysterectomy. With present inflation rates the dollar equivalent would be a few cents. Numerous friends and relatives received my services for love only.

I went to my consulting rooms and attended to patients till 11 a.m. At this time Amir and I had a standing date at the Uganda Bookshop, meeting on the second floor, where we would devour coffee and a giant sausage roll. This was a popular haunt for many, including crowds of lawyers who would come in wearing their garb, black gowns, thin ties and some even in white wigs. Amongst them we often met Aneel Korde who would later marry Laila, Amir's sister. Unabashed, we would go back to work for a brief time and then meet at home for a huge lunch. Amir then returned to work but received hot tea in a thermos and a crunchy munchy from his mother at 4 p.m., lest he starve. I stayed home with Rushna till 4 p.m., when she would be taken out to a nearby green by the ayah, and I would either schedule surgery or consult till 6 p.m. A long evening at home would then end in yet another late evening meal.

My patients were mostly Indian women with the occasional African, European or American. I drew from a solid middle of the middle class, and although my skills were rarely challenged, my Gujerati improved to the point where I almost talked 'like a native.'

The exception to my middle of middle-class clientele one day walked in happily pregnant. She had married into sugar wealth. An entire town near Kampala revolved around this business that was owned by a principal family and several lesser relatives. From miles away, the over-ripe fermented smell of sugar cane in its various stages of production could be discerned. Very different from that sweetest of nostalgic smells of coffee blossom that also grew on those long-ago soft hills

The pioneers of this family had left India and staked out this fertile land in East Africa. Soaring profits often malignantly earned were tempered by being good masters. Basic schools, clinics, and modest housing were supplied to the workers...while fortified palaces held these insular families with every imaginable luxury in

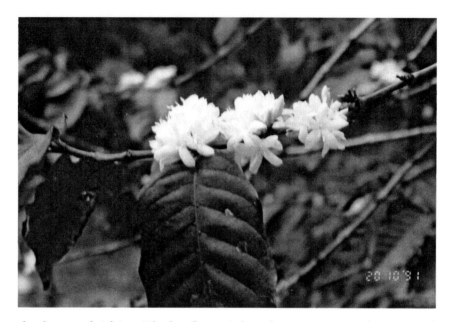

the heart of Africa. Flashy financial males, ornamented protected females, the occasional strong beauty. Overpowering in-laws were everywhere.

The patient smiled blandly through the whole encounter. I could not ask about her state of mind because of the powerful mother-in-law present at each visit. I imagined her to have been the adored exquisite daughter of a rich family in India who had been married off to a minor sugar baron. She had crossed the Indian Ocean to this continent as I had. Her body was wrapped in a fine sari, jeweled arms, onyx beaded necklace, silver tinkling anklets and sultry gold chains weighing heavily over her bare midriff. An elaborate decorated red *kum-kum* graced her forehead, declaring married, married, married. More than that—the property of those she had married.

And she was as fair and pink as a Peace rose. All this at ten in the morning, having been chauffeured in by a liveried ebon person in starchy white. What did he think as he held open the black Mercedes door for this pair? Prepare for ten years later. As you sow, so shall...

Everything seemed even and in order. I confirmed an early pregnancy, hopefully male. She swished and jingled out with all her encumbrances and beauty.

As the pregnancy progressed, she put on weight at an alarming rate. Her doe eyes receded into layers of fat, her gold belly bands had to be retired. Her elegant gold slippers were surrendered to rubber flip-flops. This was not fluid collection. It was fat. I timidly enquired into her diet. The formidable mother-in-law assured me that her diet was being looked after in the traditional vegetarian way. Ghee from home-bred cow's milk. Sweets and cheese made from the colostrums of these same over-fed cows. Excused from all her daughterly duties, she lay there and consumed what must have been a Canadian lumberjack's caloric intake. I dared say nothing to 'formidable,' reminding myself that I had always been taught there was no top limit to normal weight gain in pregnancy.

And then something else happened. At twenty-eight weeks, the uterine size measured twenty-four weeks. And there it stayed, never inching above her umbilicus. I expressed concern about this lack of fetal growth and got the reaction I feared. 'Formidable' said the solution was more calories. The mother flourished and gained seventy-five pounds in the pregnancy, but the fetus stayed at the umbilicus.

At thirty-six weeks, a motorcade transported her in labor to the nursing home. Her smile persisted throughout labor. She did not dare to express her pain, even in labor, in her mother-in-law's presence. A few grunts and she had delivered this tiny thing. She scarcely looked down. At least it was a boy. A placenta no bigger or thicker than a small *chapatti* followed.

The fragile bundle was vigorous and demanding and needed no assistance in getting on with life. A pediatric colleague declared him to be small but perfect. I saw the mother-in-law's thoughts. Somehow this was the mother's fault. Again I was relieved it was a boy.

I saw them a year later at some affair. The child was fair and smiling, replete with comfortable belly, bursting cheeks and deep creases at the braceleted ankles and amuleted wrists. A bonny overweight child well fed by grandmother. I tried not to look too hard but the mother, my patient, never lost her seventy-five pounds.

Dinner at Jacques'

Shirin, my younger sister, by now a well-established lawyer in Bombay working in the legal department of Tata—a huge corporate conglomerate—visited when Rushna was a year old. Knowing her love for good food and wine, we took her to all the available dining out there was in one-street Kampala. And one unforgettable dinner at the home of our friend Jacques.

Jacques lived in a medieval-looking mansion on one of the seven hills of Kampala. A gorgeous interior full of old painted wood carvings and ancient oils. An itchy animal skin—leopard or jaguar—sofa marred the décor. As soon as we came in the meal started. This was serious business, not to be disturbed by conversation or any such trivia. Little balls of melty pastry with some kind of matching wine started the evening.

We then entered the dining room with a huge dining table carved from a single piece of mahogany—plain and perfect. We sat around the table in King Arthur chairs waiting for the first course which, Jacques had told us repeatedly, was to be a 'light' cheese fondue. The bubbling bowl was brought in and placed in front of him. He stirred it with a fork, stared at the bowl fixedly, turned red, and exploded into a stream of French profanities which only he, who was part Belgian, and the Rwandan man waiting at the table understood. The only words that emerged clearly several times were 'chewing gum.'

When the dust settled, Jacques spluttered that he had told the cook how, if the Emmenthaler, Swiss and Gouda were left on the flame even a second longer than an expletive four minutes in the pot full of wine, Cinderella's coach would turn into a pumpkin and the cheeses would turn into chewing gum. He demonstrated long braids of thread and rope he could draw the fondue into. It looked and smelled fine to me, and I suggested we try it anyway, which further angered him. He picked up the pot and noisily emptied it into the garbage can in the kitchen. Then he flounced back and sat at his seat for all of a few seconds in pin-drop silence, then hurried back into the kitchen to supervise the next course, lest it too be destroyed. Amir, Shirin and I watched in awed silence. Such emotions over food! Out came the unbelievable next course. Four bright orange-red lobster shells containing the sweet lobster meat in a cheesy sauce (more cheese—had he just lifted the previous course out of the garbage can?), bubbling and heady with wine, speckled with herbs. A bowl of half-inch long-grain fluffy white rice followed, and some flowery wine to wash it all down.

Shirin, unmarried, was looking at Jacques, also unmarried, with distinctly suggestive eyes. This could be a marriage made in heaven at the altar of fine food and wine.

We were led back to the living room to strawberries and cream. At Shirin's questioning looks, a bottle of champagne was uncorked. Coyly Jacques asked permission to mash his strawberries into his cream, which favor he also performed for Shirin, but not Amir or me. Things were looking really promising. Next came foamy and aromatic Arabica espresso with cream that he carefully poured over the back of a spoon so as not to disturb the foam. He then brought out the Havanas, and in spite of my present stance against smoking, I can still close my eyes and remember the aroma of Arabica entwined with Havana smoke.

The denouement came a moment later when the door burst open and a young smiling black male entered. He and Jacques murmured a few quiet French love words to each other, and the lad left to go up to the bedroom.

Shirin took it quite philosophically and declared that good food was good food, and good wine was definitely good wine.

Serengeti and father

Amir and I, my year-old Rushna, and Shirin with Amir's brother Bahadur to keep her company, set out on this *safari*. We packed a few things—essential amongst them was Siu Fun's pink potty and jars of baby food. When I see the heavy machinery that my daughters (including Rushna) carry around for their children, I remember my Rushna on safari, the lightest traveler of all. And the most accommodating. She would use her potty in a speeding car on a jolting road and eat unheated food with a spoon straight out of a jar.

This was a second time for Amir and Bahadur, but Shirin, Rushna and I would see all through virgin eyes.

We crossed into Tanzania via Arusha and first visited Lake Manyara—one of the mysterious salt lakes of Africa. I imagine them connected to some ancient ocean, then getting isolated by mighty land upheavals.

This wooded park is very different from other shrubby African game country—a tropical beauty all its own. We hunted for the tree-climbing lions that the park was famous for and by the end of the day saw none. As we were leaving, we stopped for some forgotten thing and looked up to see a lioness flopped on the fork of a tree whose branches were overhanging the road. All four legs dangling amongst the branches and belly obviously distended and full, she had no interest in us.

The next day we drove to the Crater Lodge in Ngorongoro, an Eden where game is concentrated in an extinct volcanic crater. On the crater's rim we lived in cozy wood cottages heated by a fireplace and surrounded by white marguerites and Barberton daisies. Early the next morning we descended the crater in a four-wheeler for a drive of enchantment. Sleek zebras, gazelles and deer, lion prides. And rhinoceros—an impressive beast. Imagine the slaughter of this massive animal for only its horn, which is alleged to have aphrodisiac properties. And the crater lake blushing pink with

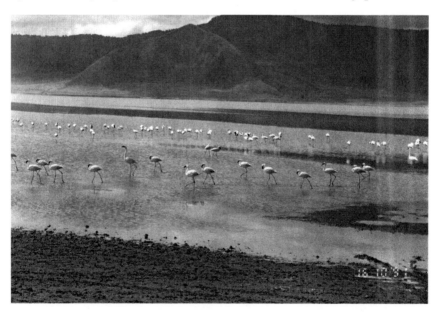

flamingos. 'Filiwingo,' Rushna called them, as do all her children.

And then on to Seronara Lodge in Serengeti. Seronara, another beautiful name I stored for future use. As we entered the park, we saw the loveliest of East African birds, the lilac-breasted roller. There were flocks of them, flying almost vertically upwards, scouting around and then diving into the grasses for some invisible delicacy.

We roamed the wild country and quietly watched lionesses at play with their cubs while a malcontent lion roamed on the periphery. A scene difficult to forget: lion family in the foreground and extended elephant family behind them, each capable of destroying the other, but living in total peace. Unforgettable to see the families sprawled and playing on the rocky outcroppings so typical of this park. As we were leaving in the dusk of evening, we saw a family, maybe a dozen lions, relaxing on a tall rock formation. We watched for a long time, Rushna unafraid and calling *simba, simba* in a soft whisper.

That night we slept in tents. And as the night quieted we started hearing the deep rumble of lions roaring, out for a night of hunting. Rushna, fearless in the day, sat bolt upright in her bed, her eyes wide with apprehension. We gathered her up and brought her into our bed and before long you would have thought the roaring lions were a lullaby.

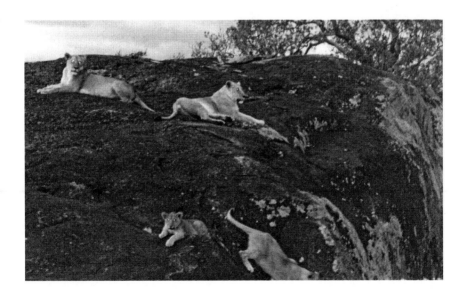

Two days after we returned, we got a call from Bombay. It was Sherry, our cousin. She told us haltingly that our Dad had died suddenly the day before. Everything stopped, congealed, blurred. 'I should never have left,' whispered Shirin, as if that would have made a difference. Nothing makes a difference.

We decided that Shirin and I would fly to Bombay. Amir found the fastest way to go would be to get a United Arab Airways flight from Nairobi to Cairo to Khartoum to Bombay. Shirin and I packed and got into the car driven by Amir and Amir, my brother-in-law. The two of them drove all night to get us to Nairobi Airport and onto our plane, and then just turned around and drove back to be on time for the next day's work.

We boarded the plane and went to the next stop, Cairo, and then on to Khartoum. A ferocious sandstorm in Khartoum kept us there for six hours. During this time, someone put on a concert of slow serious dancing, hardly dancing, just movements to wailing sad music, all by the flickering light of a giant bonfire. It was a fitting dark background to our mood. We finally made it to Bombay and were taken directly to Dungarwadi in the heart of Bombay where the Parsi Towers of Silence are located. I cannot remember ever having been to this lush and green place far away from the grime and noise of the city, with its old trees, trailing lianas and shrill calls of peacocks flying free.

As we drove up the hillside toward the *bangli* where the ceremonies are performed I saw the outline of the Tower of Silence buildings on the horizon with vultures lining the turreted tops. Although Parsis have distinguished themselves in many worlds, the thing most people know them for is the way they dispose of their dead. It is held in horror by most alien ears, but reflects a back-to-nature philosophy. The dead are bathed and wound in fine white muslin. They are laid out on a stone slab in the *bangle,* and prayers are offered for an easy passage.

On the next day, it is over, and pallbearers—consisting of a special community of people who live in small houses nearby— carry the body up to the towers and place them in circular manner open to the sun, rain and sky. When laid down the white muslin shroud is opened to expose the body, my father, to the elements. The birds of prey do the rest. 'Vulture' comes from the Latin 'vultur,' meaning 'to cleanse.' How many times in the game parks have I seen the ring of cleansers, hyena and vultures, waiting for *simba* to finish.

The pallbearers are the only people allowed into the final place in the towers. They are Parsis supported by Parsi charities. They do not leave the hill they live on. They intermarry, often incestuously, and are about four feet tall and uniformly mentally challenged. Recently Shirin told me that the city has finally got to the birds of prey, and the vulture population has dwindled, preventing them from doing the swift job they used to do. Instead of using this as a reason to change to some other form of disposal, the Parsi elders are conjuring up ways to breed and restock them.

We arrived long after my father had been taken away but sat through the three days of prayers to bid him safe and soft journey. We went home to Court View, where I had lived as a child, where I was married and where my father had lived for the last ten years of his life. And finally, decades later, this old home of ours is where Amir died suddenly one night.

I wandered into my father's room and mutely saw the depression in the cotton-filled mattress where he had slept. His white and blue shirts hanging in a polished wood cupboard. His gray suits and dark red ties.

And most painful and heartbreaking of all, his silver hair on the wooden-handled pig-bristled hairbrush he had used as far back as I can remember.

Perrin said he had the personality of water. He cleaned and refreshed but moved or changed nothing. Just passed through and left.

My father had an aluminum tumbler from his World War II days. He said he had used it for his shaving water, his drinking water, his soup and his evening *chota* peg—a generous dose of Scotch. And he had an ancient stethoscope with a bell chest piece. I brought back these two remembrances that had sustained him. The tumbler holds flowers when I remember.

Only my dearest ones back in Africa could hold me. I flew back as soon as I could, to Amir and Rushna.

1965: Pica

One day Ma confided in me her *pica*—uncontrollable urge to eat what is not commonly considered edible—urge to eat clay while pregnant.

She told me that with each pregnancy she had an overwhelming desire not to eat just any clay, but clay she found on the lonely bank of a river that ran through Sultanhamud and another in Singida. Even now, in menopause, she talked of it longingly and said that if she were transported back to those places, she would head for that favorite spot and glory in that long-ago taste.

She said the clay she favored was fine and white and had body. It was sweetish and bland and felt like *malaii*—heavy cream on the tongue—like plain white rice, flat baked bread or steamed *matoke*—comfort foods. She smiled and said that she jealously guarded this secret spot, not from a reluctance to reveal her longings—she knew other women had their favorite spots—but so that she could keep this precious piece of earth to herself.

I asked her how she ate at her secret spot. Just go there and gouge it out and consume? Impossible. She was a delicate eater. Like most Asian women of her time, she ate with her well-washed hands, forming small tasty balls on her right index, middle fingers and thumb, and propelling them into her mouth with a subtle twist of her thumb. Eating with one's fingers is an art. Some can do it flickeringly and only involve the tips of three fingers. Others have to roll up their sleeves and have liquid flowing down to their elbows which has to be licked and sucked and slurped to prevent everything from being stained a golden oily tumeric yellow. Ellis, my oldest grandchild, preferentially eats with his fingers—unfortunately not as delicately as Ma. A genetic throwback, his mother claims.

Ma, the artful eater, looked surprised at the question. She said she carried a tiny clay (more clay, more lead) saucer and spoon to the spot. Once she confirmed she was unobserved, she dug up a small spoonful to taste. Some areas were too salty, and she would move and sample till she got it just right. She would shape the clay into a little ball—like an ice-cream scoop. Sometimes she brought along some well water and let it run through the clay, drain it, then reshape it and enjoy.

What creates this urge? Does anemia cause it, or does it result from the clay preventing iron absorption, and the lead in the clay further poisoning the blood-forming cells?

Decades later, a pale and pasty Hispanic woman walked into my office in New York. She was overtly anemic—third-world anemia and astronomical serum lead levels. Through an interpreter and with much prodding she described her decrepit apartment, complete with ferocious landlord who refused to paint peeling walls and replace corroded pipes. By now all in the room were rallying against the prototype of the vicious uncaring landlord. Clearly the woman needed to be removed from her environment, and the child she lived with needed to be tested. She was admitted to hospital. Social Services investigated her home and brought the child for testing. There was no evidence of exposed lead in the home, and the child's lead levels were in the normal range.

When questioned again, she hinted at pica, and when further encouraged, she stated that she regularly ate clay in this and all of her previous four pregnancies.

Hydration, treatment with agents that leached out the lead and supplemental iron soon brought her back.

Another woman guarding her pica urge.

Rushna goes to school

At the ripe old age of two, Rushna was enrolled into Mrs. Jones' School—never dignified by a formal name. Rushna met her milestones at an accelerated rate—to put it modestly. At nine months, when she had lived an equal span of life within and without the womb, she said her first word. Not adoring mama or dada, but 'outside.' She evidently thought this was a good solution for all tensions. With the friendly equable weather of Kampala, 'outside' was always possible. Although in theory we had a short rain and a long rain, in actuality each day had a little sun, a little rain, a little this and a little that, always hovering around a glorious 75 degrees. I dread to think of a dead-of-winter 'outside' North American baby.

I can hardly remember when Rushna was not potty trained, and Siu Fun's pink potty was her favorite. One day on a weekday when we were home for lunch and sitting across from each other in the tiny living room, Rushna, all of ten months old, was standing next to me and just decided to walk over to Amir. Just as he walked on air when she was born, he sang to himself, 'Shadlu chali, shadlu chali'—'She walked, she walked.' And there he was, walking on air again. So Rushna walked at ten months and read at two years, but I have to add that she rebelled and tore our hearts in an alien space at sixteen and then returned and befriended me at twenty-one. And ever after.

One day back when she was a toddler I gave her a tiny sturgeon egg that she licked off my finger. The next day I asked her what she wanted for dinner and she said 'cabiar.' Enough, we thought, she is ready for school.

So on the appointed day I drove her to Mrs. Jones' School which Mrs. Ginny Jones had started in the spacious garage of her hillside home. She was young, energetic and enthusiastic, but it was impossibly difficult to leave Rushna. I drew it out till Mrs. Jones practically threw me out. I walked down the driveway, and then something made me turn and I saw Rushna's dark serious dry large painful eyes on me. I left, but only after she had imprinted her eyes on my heart. It was a memorable event—the beginning of long years of learning. The beginnings of the fastest and most prolific reader there ever was. The beginnings of a facile understanding and a liberal heart.

School was a success, and she stopped giving me the dark eye when I left.

FIVE

Roscoe Road and Cena

15-17 Roscoe Road and Cena

Later that year, the landlord, an Ismaili who rented us our Baskerville Avenue house, paid us a visit. As far as we could tell, without provocation, he warned us to mend our messy ways, specially as our neighbors were white, an insult we were too angry to respond to, but one that motivated us to look for a plot of land and build. Perhaps that was just what the landlord wanted — to increase the rent without a hassle from us.

We found an acre-sized plot a short walk from our present hours at Roscoe Road, and in 1965 we started to build the home we lived in till we left Kampala in 1971.

The land was fronted by Roscoe Road and a green beyond, which was later the site for a Government secondary school. To the right was Lower Kololo Terrace Road that curved around the foot of Kololo Hill. Beyond this was the Hindu crematorium. The trees in the crematorium were always festooned by icy-eyed Maribou storks that had no fear and could be stared at from close by. Much after we had left, someone wrote that these giant storks were all over the city, feeding on uncollected garbage as the city deteriorated under Amin. To our left was a stand of fragrant eucalyptus trees, a long-ago import from Australia, whispering in the soft breeze.

We used a pair of young Ismaili architects who had never done anything before. Amir's requirement was that it be a ranch house. I, too, preferred children at the same level we were at all times. So we built this house with Amir literally carrying most of the materials to the site in the back of his German car, a two-toned blue Opal.

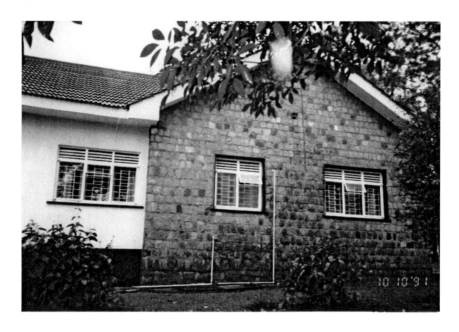

On the front of the red-tiled verandah, an almost carnivorous alamanda creeper later grew with tentacles turned houseward each morning, no matter how we hacked it away during the day. In my home in Ossining, there is a wisteria with similar tendencies growing up from the porch into our bedroom. Periodic hacking keeps it at bay. A living room ran the full length of the house with a warm parquet floor. A dining room making an L with the living room held a democratic round table we bought from an ailing British woman whose yellow eyes could not wait to leave the country. The kitchen had white cabinets and a spotted terrazzo floor. A wing of bedrooms on the other side of the living room made a C shape enclosing a stone-tiled courtyard with plants and vines, where we spent long and lovely hours.

And to my present shame, there was a small detached house for the domestic help: small rooms, single lightbulbs and a common toilet at some distance from our house with—too horrible to tell—a bell that could be rung from the house whenever we wished to summon them. It is the memory of this that makes me understand the power of falling in with whatever is the pattern of life. Yet there were others who did not. I remember Dr. Gerry Shaper, who had been my consultant during my Internal Medicine rotation, saying that he and his wife did not and would never employ domestic help. I can hardly get myself to call them what we did at the time— servants.

And yet we did. Most around us justified it by saying we were providing employment, but I knew better. It was a form of employment that imprisoned and crippled. Why should anyone earn a living by washing someone else's dirty underwear, supplying food, cleaning?

But that is what happened. There was Elena, a young beautiful woman who was fun and laughing. She taught all my children Swahili as the first language they spoke, and often they would prattle to each other in that language before they became fluent in British-accented English, picked up by Rushna in her school and transferred to her sisters. Years later in 1971 when we found ourselves in Brooklyn, Swahili was rapidly forgotten—hopefully it still lurks in some forgotten gyri—and the most appalling Brooklyn English took its place. Later still, and to this day, they speak American-accented English, which locals tell me is 'English with no accent.' We also employed Ramzani, a distinguished-looking tall Moslem who helped himself handily to the supplies in the house— all except, because he was a Moslem, alcohol. His young school-going daughter lived with him. Ramzani was the head of that level of the household and arbitrated all the petty stuff.

Once when I asked why his meat curries always turned out so different, he said, 'Cooking is like gambling—sometimes you win and sometimes you lose.' He spoke impeccable coastal Swahili and tolerated my massacring the language. He knew I reversed *funga* and *fungua*—close and open—and did the opposite of what I said, until Amir insisted on correcting me when all understanding broke down and Ramzani was closing up when I asked him to open.

And then there was Leopold, the gardener from the Congo. He was a virile, silent Mellors-type straight from D.H. Lawrence's *Chatterley* who soon was in the throes of a romance with Elena which she later wanted out of. Ramzani solved this tangle in some magical way that brought them back to being just friends.

By August of 1965, I developed my violent aversion for alcohol, which confirmed I was pregnant. And on Christmas Day, we

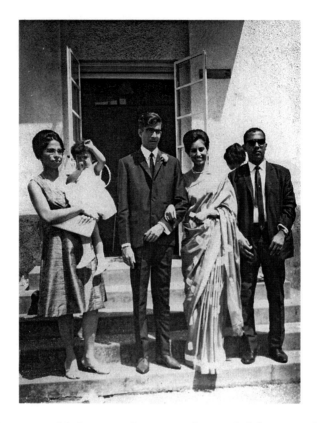

moved into our shining new house, so beautiful that I could barely manage to leave it for daily activities. The living room had a long wall of glass doors opening into the verandah. I covered that wall with a massive curtain the color of the rift valley. Or so my vanity thought. Faded gold.

In February of 1966 Amir's sister Laila married our lawyer friend Aneel, Laila an Ismaili and Moslem and Aneel a Hindu, sworn enemies on another stage. But the elders in both families were enlightened and progressive, and Aneel and Laila were not observant, so all was celebratory.

There were days of celebration, including a Chinese meal at our home. Sweet and sour pork was on the menu, and I suddenly looked around and saw Ma's friends, a group of Ismaili ladies, tucking into the dish and exclaiming how delicious the *bhajias* were.

Being observant Moslems, they had sworn never to touch pork, but it was too late. I just turned away and let them sin in peace. A barrel full of ice and myriad cooling champagne bottles kept our guests well supplied. I took a rain check on that. I had to attend a delivery on the night before the wedding and literally went home in the morning, showered, donned a grey silk maternity dress, went to Gulpar, the hair dresser, who backcombed my hair into a beehive that was the fashion of the day, and drove over to City Hall for the civil ceremony. Photographs of the bridal couple show an exquisite Laila in a yellow and green sari and handsome slim dark-suited Aneel.

This time I went to Dr. Trussell for my pregnancy, as Dr. Kayton had gone back to the U.K. All went well and a merciful median episiotomy resulted in this smallest of all my babies, who latched onto the breast like a charm and was a voracious eater. Amir named her Cena after a friend's child, Sheena. On a trip to Spain when Cena was ten years old, she marveled at her fame when all the dinner menus had Cena written on them.

When we brought her home, I wanted Rushna to take part in child care to avoid competition and jealousy. In those days, Baby Johnson talcum powder was used in lavish quantities and in the first hour that Cena was home, Rushna managed to get a blob of it in the baby's wide open eye, instead of her petal-smooth bottom. It was a strange and unforgettable thing to see Cena, wide-eyed and uncrying, with a ball of powder in her eye. I checked my hysteria and rubbed it away.

1966: Royalty

I was back to work in my practice when one day I was hand-delivered a letter requiring me to attend to the *Nabagereka*, the official wife of the Kabaka and Queen of Buganda. I was given no details, but was told to appear at the palace in the old part of the town at four that afternoon. I cancelled my consultation schedule for the afternoon and presented my royal letter at the gun-guarded gate at a few minutes before four, and after some discussion in which I had no part, I was waved in.

I entered an airy room and was told that she, the *Nabagereka*

Damali Kisankole, would be with me presently. Someone had warned me to anticipate a prolonged wait and I had taken along a newspaper. Two hours later, as I was fretting about my children and feeling my breasts tingle with the need to feed Cena, she entered—an utterly regal figure in cool western dress, panty hose and high heels. Quiet, beautiful and smiling. I had previously seen the *Kabaka*'s favorite wife, Sara Kisankole, who was Damali's sister. Sara was a hefty bouncing woman, quite unlike this serene Queen. Bapa used to say *'Rajane gamti rani,'*—'the queen is whom the king prefers.' And it ended *'chhane vinte ani'*—'no matter if she handles the cow dung.' The heart cannot be questioned and gives no answers.

I had also been warned never to appear physically taller than Baganda royalty. Attendants in the room came in, advanced and shuffled around on their knees so as to achieve this. Out of consideration for me, the queen remained standing and instructed me to remain seated. I was construing how a gynecologic examination could be achieved with this restriction but I need not have worried because she had no intention of being examined by me.

After she had asked after my health and that of my family, and after an attendant had shuffled in on her knees with my favorite milky *chai*, she said she had a problem. A female problem. She spoke of her vaginal discharge as troublesome and irritating in the third person—as though it was happening to someone else. I was rapidly disoriented and asked questions like, 'Does she have a discharge with a bad odor?' Both of us were unwilling to admit that the queen had this commoner's problem. It turned out that her discharge was white, curdy, odorless and irritating.

I timidly suggested that I examine the patient, whoever she may be. I had brought along gloves, speculum and flashlight. I was rebuked and told that she had a regular gynecologist, someone whom she trusted (as opposed to me), and who had delivered her children and collected her Pap smears. She named a great white icon as her gynecologic attendant.

In my code, I had never treated a patient without a physical examination. Where should I go? This was clearly what she was asking me to do. My predicament did not last long. She kindly told me that I was to prescribe a cure and if 'the patient' did not feel better she would get herself examined by her regular gynecologist. In a flash I compromised years of old teaching, common sense and expediency triumphing over principle. I brought out my prescription pad and prescribed Mycostatin vaginal suppositories for what seemed to be a yeast infection. Hesitatingly I wrote Queen Damali's name, since we had never clearly established who the patient was, hoping that this would not offend her. Thoughts of whether she could be harboring 'something else' clouded my imminent escape. I gulped and trusted that she did not have a worse infection or even cancer. I could see the Uganda Argus headlines, 'Incompetent Indian Doc misses cervix cancer in Damali, Queen of Buganda.'

I handed the prescription to the Queen, stressing that the medication should only be used by 'the patient' vaginally. I was then dismissed, but was careful not to stand before she left. I held back the impulse to tell her what my modest fee was. Why was I so easily repressed by royalty? Old hang-ups surface. I had been twice colonized and easy to overpower.

I escaped to my fold. Where had you been? To Mengo to see the Queen. And, pussycat, what did you do there? I frightened a little mouse under a chair. Regrettably, I did not even dare to do that.

Encounter at gunpoint

Meanwhile things were far from tranquil politically. Obote and his Colonel Amin were accused of misappropriating funds intended for the Congo. There were also rumors of their participation in gold and ivory smuggling from the same country. To the rising cries of disapproval, Obote suppressed all opposition parties, and Uganda was fast becoming a one-party state with no hope of elections. The newspapers rapidly became a mouthpiece of the government.

One afternoon Amir, Rushna, Cena and I went to Mengo, the old part of the city, to visit Amir's aunt and show her the new baby. On our way home I was driving, Amir was in the passenger seat with Cena in his arms, and Rushna was in the back seat. We were suddenly surrounded by hyper-excited militia who crowded our car. One of them poked a weapon through the passenger-seat window and demanded to know what we were doing here when there was a war on. He was excited and spewing saliva as he barked at us. We did not dare to ask what war he was talking about. In a fit of generosity he said '*Toka, toka*' barking at me to drive away fast. That's just what I did.

We seemed to live with an inexplicable tolerance for danger. Although our children and our lives had been recently threatened, I remember no fear. We almost expected to be surrounded by violence and yet continue with our lives as though all this had little to do with us. Impossible to explain.

When we got home, we heard that Obote, wanting to consolidate his position, had ousted the Kabaka, King of the Baganda, earlier that that day. Amin had stormed the palace and taken it over. The Kabaka, it was rumored, dressed as a woman, escaped under the confusion of a thunderstorm, eventually to Britain where he died in 1969, a chronic alcoholic with a strangely weak but noble Bantu face.

1967: Curfew, race and the Memvuwalla

The Baganda, whose King had been removed both from an ancient inherited monarchy and from the presidency of the country, were outraged and marginalized. Things were further fragmented by infighting in Obote's UPC party with a breakaway wing being led by Grace Ibingira, the Minister of Justice, who represented the Bantu peoples and was supported by the Baganda against Obote's northerners.

A dusk-to-dawn curfew was imposed on us. Dusk was a vague term, but fell suddenly in this equatorial country, and no one wanted to challenge the exact time. So we were all home and indoors by 7 p.m. Unfortunately, Cena had a need for fresh air, and Amir used to walk her up and down a brick path leading from the house to the 'down garden' to put her to sleep. He declared that she, Cena, aged all of nine months, insisted that this ritual continue. So baby Cena, who had recently had a rifle pointed at her, was walked up and down the brick path while her father crooned a tuneless song that he had created for her about cool, cool breezes. The next word in the song was '*khaye.*' Translated literally, it meant 'we will eat the cool, cool breezes.' In Gujerati 'eat' was often used for 'feel' or 'experience,' a telling insight into our personalities. While outside defying the curfew, he said that whenever a car passed lower Kololo Terrace, which was the main road that swept around our corner plot of land, he would duck, baby in arms, into the bushes to avoid the headlights. What were we thinking? We were thirty-three years of age and in spite of the violence around us, fear of death never entered into our still secure world.

Being in solo practice, I did a lot of night work and had to drive during curfew hours. Doctors' cars were identified by plates added to the front and back fenders that were supposed to protect us. As I write, I can see mounting catastrophe, but in the midst of it, we felt nothing of this. We were amazingly secure and trusting in our Uganda citizenship and papers, which we never questioned would establish us as Ugandans and therefore belonging. We underestimated the power of race and color to set people apart— and tribe and religion.

I should have seen it all around me. We professed being Ugandan first. But the only black Africans who entered our house on a regular basis were the people who did menial jobs for us. Ma (my mother-in-law) professed no such Ugandan feelings and would, to Amir's and my protests, use derogatory terms to address the black African.

And yet there was a tall man, an ancient man with a gaunt face and Arab features, who would rap at Ma's back *sakati* carrying a basket of little yellow Uganda bananas, pineapples and home-grown vegetables. The *memvuwalla*—banana seller. After bargaining over a bunch or two of bananas, she would draw up two stools and they would quietly converse in coastal Swahili. They often passed a whole afternoon in conversation, each loving the pure Swahili spoken by so few people in this land-locked country. She, born in the coastal Arab-influenced island of Lamu in Kenya, and he from some long forgotten Arab-African ancestry.

We often asked what they talked of. '*Sukh dukh ni vat,*' she would say. 'We talked of happiness and sorrow.' None of us who professed belonging to the country had such a quiet friendship with an African black.

And this same Ma, years before I knew her, in Singida had

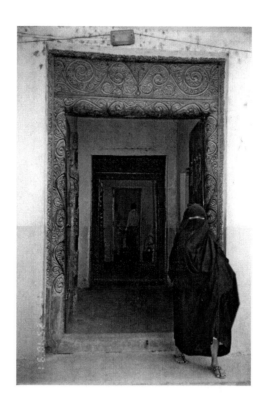

coined a phrase that we use to this day. '*Hapana kabila yetu,*'—'not of our kind.' A neighbor, an Ith-na-ashari Moslem (as opposed to the Ismaili Moslem that she was), had guests and needed extra seating. He came to Ma's door and asked for the *bhenkro*—the bench she had in her *sakati*. She refused to lend the bench to him, citing, '*Hapana kabila yetu*' as the reason. Years later in the U.S., she was reminiscing and said that there were only a few things she regretted in her life, things that she felt she would eventually have to answer for, and this was one of them.

Bahadur, who was an English major at the local Makerere University, played among the intellectual elite of Uganda. I watched him trying too hard. He often brought his colleagues to my home, and I imagined myself as a latter-day Gertrude Stein, fostering these people who lived for writing and thinking. I never was invited back to their houses. That should have told the story. The truth was never far from the surface, and on one occasion

Bahadur had annoyed all by lowering the volume of the music and dimming the bright lights as was his life-long habit. One of the crowd wanted Bahadur's jacket to tie around his waist so he could perform the traditional *dingi-dingi* dance. Bahadur refused, and the playwright Robert Serumaga accused him of being a racist, telling him with intended cruelty that he could never be black no matter how hard he tried. A bitter lesson.

On one occasion way before I had my children, Bahadur brought Mugoro, a Makerere student, home to Ma's house. Mugoro had been brought because we were going on a camping trip and he was to lend us a tent large enough to accommodate nine of us. There was a grassy space behind Ma's house where Mugoro put us all to work. This was no pop-up nylon tent. It was heavy canvas with poles and pegs and guy ropes that had to be pulled with discipline and split-second timing. Finally, at the end of three hours of training, Mugoro was satisfied that we more or less knew what we were doing and entrusted us with his tent. We came in and had a meal. As it was late, Bahadur suggested Mugoro sleep over at Ma's house. He was given a room and left his dusty boots outside his door, evidently expecting them to be polished. The houseboy next day told Ma that he had brought Mugoro a drink, cleared away his dishes, made a bed for him, but would never, never, ever polish his shoes.

SIX

Sharyn

1968: Sharyn

We were planning on a third baby, but it happened sooner than we thought. A contraceptive failure in May soon gave me the familiar 'can't stand alcohol' sign and we knew Sharyn was conceived. Amir always chuckled and called her '*Bhul*' Tejani—mistake Tejani—and then would add, 'the best mistake we ever made.' Because of this dear accident, she was three years old when we left for the U.S. Had the accident not occurred, she would have been much younger, and we might have postponed our plans for emigration—and then would have been forced out a year later by Idi Amin. Most fortunate of accidents!

I was due in February 1968, but we fitted in a holiday to Mombasa in January when I was hugely pregnant.

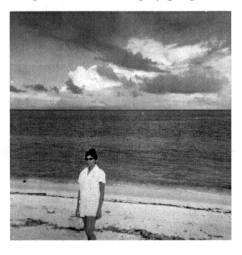

We rented a cottage on the beach in Bamburi and sent our entourage, Elena and Ramzani, by train and followed by car. We cooked and ate and swam and played. We bought fish at Amir's cousin's fish store, the same cousin who had taken me to secret grottos when I had first arrived. Only now he would say he had reserved the freshest fish for me at a special price. Special it was— twice as expensive as elsewhere. Our friends Piroja—as pregnant as I and whose baby I was to deliver a few weeks later—and Feredun Amrolia, pillars of the Parsi community in Kampala, were also in Mombasa with Shirish and Rashmi Clerk. Shirish was to serendipitously deliver the baby I was carrying at the time. Musical chairs.

There was a coral reef just beyond the beach outside our cottage. The tides in Mombasa were dramatic. At high tide all would be covered, and at low tide the water would be so far out that one could walk on parts of the reef. I liked to time it when the reef was two or three feet deep and I would spend hours out there, snooping on water life. Sparkling sunlight in the clear waters guided my way to sea anemones waving their fronds with saffron and black clownfish playing inside them. There were parrot fish the color of peacocks, angel fish and the occasional manta ray undulating on the ocean floor. And then the coral—fire and brain, staghorn and fossil. And echinodermata, five fingered star-fish of every hue and description. On earlier trips I had dived and brought out treasures from the sea which quickly lost their sparkle on land. My pregnancy stopped me from this massacre, and I never again touched what I saw underwater.

Sometimes the water I snorkeled in was so shallow that I had to hold my pregnant belly in with my hands to protect Sharyn. On one occasion I emerged from the ocean to see Piroja and some Parsi friends she had attracted staring at my pregnant self as I came out. 'Marere,' they said, 'is it safe to do this in your condition?'

The pregnancy swimsuit I wore was comical--a brightly colored flowery affair consisting of a pair of enormous bloomers and a mini dress to modestly cover them. Very different from the enchanting suits I see on the beach today--bikinis with the swollen belly held out for all to admire between the bra and pants.

The coral reef was also full of live and fossil sea urchins. One day, my pregnancy making me less well balanced in water, my foot landed heavily on a live sea urchin with enormous black bristles. The bristles penetrated my flippers and pierced the sole of my foot, causing a painful chemical reaction. I got myself out of the ocean and dragged over to the cottage in awful pain. A few hours later an ancient man came to the cottage and said he had heard that a pregnant woman had a sea urchin injury and he had a cure. Amir almost drove him away, but I made him stay. He showed me a dirty rag in which there were several pieces of the magic remedy. Raw papaya was one, and the others were unrecognizable. Since the pain was awful and there appeared to be no other remedy, I did what he said and let him tie the rag around my foot to apply the magic stuff to the injured area. He did this slowly and thoughtfully, all the time singing a high-pitched incantation which was part of the cure. An hour later the pain had vanished, and I was ready to snorkel again.

We were back in Kampala a few weeks before I was due. In the middle of February I delivered Laila, Amir's sister, of her first born, Rukesh. Rukesh and Sharyn were babies together, often sharing the bathtub, cousins and good friends to this day—and both lawyers in Washington D.C. A few days after Rukesh was born, on the

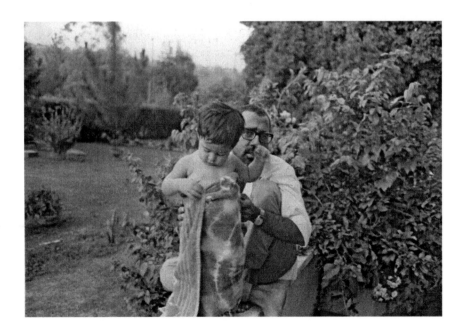

night of 25th of February, I went into labor myself. The labor was as excruciating as always but fast, and I was fully dilated by 8 a.m. on the 26th. There was no sign of the obstetrician, Dr. Trussell, but my old friend Shirish Clerk happened to be passing by and was corralled in to help. Thinking I would be upset to have yet another girl, I remember him announcing her birth by saying, 'The three graces.' And I reassured him by saying I never expected anything but a girl. Sharyn with dark long bristly hair, 'the wrong end of a broomstick,' a friend said, and long sweeping eyelashes with sculpted arch eyebrows and curvy lips. Such a decorated face.

Ma visited me in hospital and tried to convey her sorrow at no sons for her darling Amir. I always felt that Ma had a formidable intellect and given different circumstances would have excelled at anything she put her mind to. I therefore sat her down and explained to her, in my now much-improved Gujerati, the genetics of sex determination and how I just waited passively with my X chromosomes while Amir seemed unable to supply the requisite Y chromosome. She never discussed the matter with me again.

The day we brought Sharyn home she started projectile vomiting. After a week of this, Amir called a friend/pediatrician Peter Debuse home to ask for advice. Sharyn appeared bonny and well and was gaining weight, lending no support to my story. Finally he asked me to feed her in his presence. Shedding all modesty in the interest of motherly concern, I fed her in my bedroom with Peter hovering inches away from my bared breast, ostensibly to pick out any fault in my feeding technique. That feeding, the little menace happily slurped and ate, contentedly burping and falling off to sleep soon after, the problem miraculously and permanently cured.

Market and garden

I started to visit the local Nakasero market every week. Every Saturday ladies from the villages would come into town and set up their small stalls of produce. The woman in the first stall was heavyset, quiet, and carried herself like some ancient African queen complete with gorgeous headdress. She sat behind her home-grown, irregularly sized tomatoes, cucumbers and carrots, hardly looking up from the crochet work she was always busy with.

Unlike the others, she never bargained, and if some disrespectful customer tried, she did not answer to let known her scorn. Once I put a whole lot of her produce in my cloth bag and realized I had forgotten my money. I started to put the vegetables back, but she leaned over, held my hand and said quietly, 'Next week.' The dignity and generosity of the poor.

The market was on a sharply inclined hill, and on one occasion I was walking back to my car behind a man wheeling a cart full of small tart green yellow Ugandan oranges. He tripped and lost his hold on the cart, which upturned, and for a few moments there were swirling oranges all over the inclined road. As he scurried to retrieve what he could, there materialized from every corner urchins who deftly fielded and pocketed whatever they could. A quick sharp ballet, and in a few moments there was only a crying man left on stage. Later, as I described the scene to a friend, she said that the urchins used to plant a rock on the hill to cause this accident and enable unpunishable robbery.

The meat market was behind the vegetable market, and I would avoid going there. Freshly slaughtered goat meat was used by all, as the beef was of stringy quality. These delicate goat shanks and sides liberally covered with flies hung on old blood-encrusted hooks. Cooking killed all the potential problems, but...

And the chickens. We ate roosters and not hens—the opposite of India, where we ate the female. Each claimed they ate the more tender bird. I think that in Africa they maintained the hens for eggs and got rid of the useless cocks. As you wended your way through the chicken market, you realized the origin of the expression 'chicken with its head cut off.' The unfortunate would have its head sliced off in one stroke of a *panga* and then be allowed to perform a final wild headless death dance. The seller then plucked the bird, and with a few well-aimed sweeps of his hand, cleaned it of its innards which were thrown on a huge communal heap that was later cleaned off by stray dogs and the dramatic Maribou storks that roamed the city. And then, with the sharpest of knives, the seller quartered the bird and wrapped it all in newspaper. The rest was up to you.

Garden

We had an acre of land around our house, a corner plot between lower Kololo Terrace and Roscoe Road. It was newly developed land and full of life. Even the supporting stakes we stuck in the ground would leaf out. The day we broke ground we had a small ceremony and buried what we thought were symbolic and personally important things under what was to be a supporting wall in the living room. I have heard of people agonizing over what to pack in Voyager spaceships destined for outer space. Clearly they had a more daunting task than mine, having to represent the human race to any intelligent life they might meet. What language would they use to express us? I recall they decided on some universally true mathematical equations, Jimmy Carter's flat tones on a tape, and a Bach fugue played by the enigmatic Canadian pianist Glenn Gould to express symmetry in music. Why were there no pictures of the blue and green earth with invitations and directions to visit?

We buried a copy of the *Uganda Argus* for that day, some representative Ugandan coins, typical being the now-useless one cent coin with a hole in its center, with rice and rose petals in a clay jar, a copy of a book whose title I am amazed not to remember, and a picture of Amir, Rushna and me pregnant with Cena.

Much before the house was even started we planted an evergreen hedge over the pole and chicken-wire fence that staked out what was ours, we thought, forever. The house was on a slight elevation and on the incline that surrounded the house we planted myriads of magenta, orange and butter-yellow portulacae that opened with the morning and closed at sundown, obedient to the curfew. The rest of the garden I left till we had moved.

This garden is fresh in my memory because in 1991 we went back to visit and it still existed as it had been planted. We went to Kampala in 1991 with the specific purpose of visiting our old home. Before we left we had sold it to an African assessor, Mr. Kataramu. We heard later that Kataramu had survived the Amin years, but one day answered a knock at the front door and was shot at our doorstep by *kondos*—burglars—who left him to die while they ransacked the house. When we contacted Mrs. Kataramu in 1991 telling her we wanted to see the house she was very nervous and

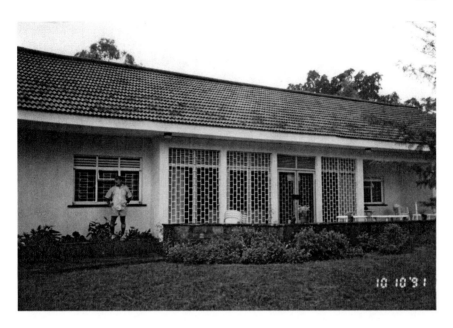

refused, as this was a time when many Asians were returning to claim old properties seized in the Idi Amin years. We assured her this was not the case but she was still reluctant and told us to ask the present renter's permission. It was rented to some minor dignitary in the British Embassy. We walked into the British Embassy and after much ado were given permission only to walk outside in the garden and not enter the house.

So the next day at nine in the morning our taxi driver Badru took us there. I could hardly see anything for my tears, and then while in the garden a heavy storm with rain and thunder suddenly played out. The ayah and houseboy took pity on us and invited us in out of the storm. We explained our purpose, and these humble folk sympathized and were kind enough to let us wander the old home where we had lived and laughed and had our children.

The garden seemed to divide itself out into a front garden, a round garden at the side of the house, a down garden at the corner farthest from the house and a back garden for fruit trees, vegetables and a playground.

We screened the front garden from the driveway with a perennial poinsettia hedge.

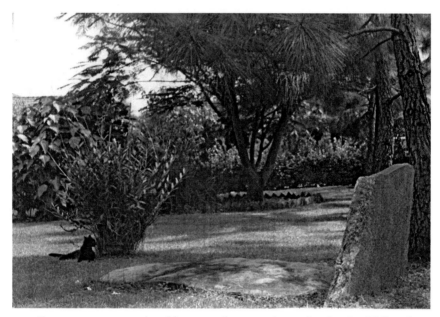

I can never get myself to purchase poinsettias in the U.S. when I remember those human height specimens. We planted a row of pines along the inside of the hedge. Thirty years later, they were more than forty feet high.

Within the front garden, I had two stones, one large and flat and the other vertical, at right angles to it. 'A tombstone,' Amir would tease, but it served for sitting and playing on. In the middle of the front garden was a rectangular-shaped three-foot-deep lily pond, which was home to hardy pink water lilies we had picked from the wild, and also papyrus from the banks of the Nile. The Paleozoic slime at the bottom of the pond became home to swirling tadpoles and some fat toads. One afternoon Rushna had a friend over and was collecting tadpoles in a jar, and Cena tried to help. Her nice little rotund frame overbalanced, and she fell into this frog-infested muddy pool. I was right there and fished her out. The tears eventually stopped, but she refused to go anywhere near water after that and would not bathe for weeks. Luckily she recovered and is today a smooth swimmer.

The round garden at the side of the house was edged in stone. The circular bed it contained was filled with roses. Sharyn was irresistibly attracted to the fat pink sweet-scented cabbage roses, and

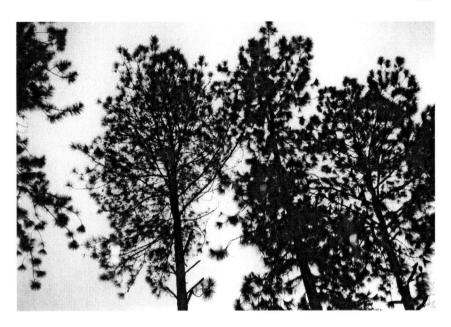

I would catch her with her mouth full of rose petals or betrayed by her rose breath. The round garden was entered between two small trees that flowered pink like cherry trees, perfect for climbing, and I would often find Rushna sprawled in the branches like a Manyara tree-climbing lion.

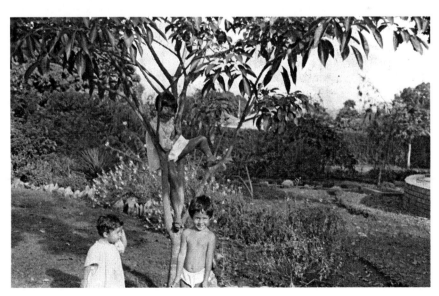

Then there was the down garden. You walked to it over a brick pathway with bottlebrush trees lining the sides. These, too, are now full grown and lovely, edged with bottlebrush flowers like scarlet painted nails. The down garden was square and had a purple flowering potato tree in the center. This tree grows rapidly and was fully grown in a couple of years. This garden had beds along the side that were planted with tropical annuals and perennials. Annuals were difficult to discern from perennials as they lasted much longer than their name suggested. Nasturtiums sprawling all over were and are my favorite. I now grow them as a vegetable and eat the flowers and round dew-dropped leaves. Their strange and typical odor always remind me of Rushna playing in this, her secret garden. Blue-sky morning glories twirled around sprouting stakes. Marigolds and marguerites decorated each other. Phlox, short and colorful, but odorless unlike those in the temperate zone. And all enhanced by bushes of fragrant *ratki-rani*, queen-of-the-night, that unleashed knee-weakening perfume after curfew hours. I jumbled all the colors together and never even thought that great gardens were made by thought to design and color. No elegant white gardens for me.

In the back garden we planted several papaya trees from seeds of fruit we had eaten. We then retained one male and three females which gave us fruit in two years. It really pains me to pay dollars for a miserable papaya today when in my Kampala garden I just plucked sweet ones right from the female tree. We also planted an avocado which we never saw fruit but was in full fruit on our return visit in 1991. Most evocative of all, I had planted a clump of lemon grass, a tea flavoring I have used from childhood and still do. Thirty years later the clump was luxuriant and green and fresh with that nostalgic smell. The present occupants of the house could not have the slightest idea of what this clump was and how it can be used to make the tea of kings and queens.

Elena, Ramzani and Leopold planted several *matoke* trees, which soon gave them their daily staple and us the occasional luxury. My children would go to them almost daily to share *matoke* steamed in banana leaves with peanut sauce.

A slide, swing and monkey bars completed the back garden.

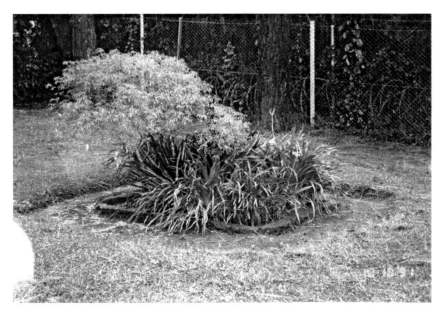

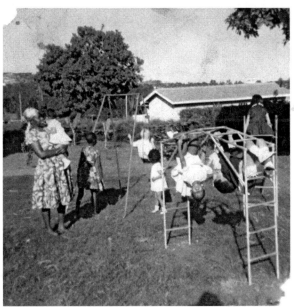

Three mature mango trees that satisfied my yen for raw mangos with salt and chilli powder also graced our garden. I buried the umbilical cord stumps of Cena and then Sharyn under one of these, and it would not stop flowering and fruiting. Some years later when a secondary school was built opposite our house I could not keep the children away from the tree, all thronging to share the mangos. A joyous sight is a mango tree in blossom whose heavy musky smell remains in the heart. *Mohur*, it is called in Gujerati, meaning 'like a peacock.'

Fistula sisters

I was sitting in the living room gazing at baby Sharyn when the telephone rang. It was my friend Piroja. They've killed him, she said. Robert Kennedy, joining the presidential race, had been shot in California. How can anyone believe that the course of life cannot be changed by one person? The U.S. we live in today would have been on a different plane if the Kennedys had lived out their lives. And, earlier that year, Dr. Martin Luther King, also felled by a wild man's hand.

Asians in Uganda were getting anxious about their future in the country. Many, being British citizens of a second-class sort, had started probing possibilities in England and Canada. Amir and I did not think we would leave, but after the indignities of having spent much of our lives colonized, we vowed that if we had to, it would not be England. This despite the fact that our credentials and my specialization were recognized in England, thus not requiring any further qualification or tests. We toyed with the idea of the U.S., but the recent assassinations there made us uneasy. So did the escalating involvement in Viet Nam. Our discussions often ended with a Scarlet-like, 'We'll think of it in the morning.'

Almost immediately after I heard of Robert Kennedy's death I got a call from Dr. Andresson, an Icelandic surgeon in his eighties who also used the small hospital I attended. He knew I was chafing at the bland day-after-day practice I had and asked me to see him that evening as he had something exciting to tell me.

And this was the story:

A Belgian missionary doctor from Butare, Rwanda, had arrived in Kampala. Basic clothes, no make-up. She was that type. Following her were seven women walking with legs tightly pressed together to minimize leakage—the fistula shuffle.

The proximity of bladder to vagina is a piece of cruel anatomy, just a sheet of tissue separating them. Women laboring for long hours face an obstructed catastrophe, an impasse with the baby long dead with its head pressing on that fragile septum, causing its dissolution. Long labor, dead birth, stormy febrile days to follow and then uncontrollable urine loss through the vagina—a common sad tale.

A foul uriniferous smell and leakage cause these women to be abandoned by man and family. They find each other and live together. Fistula sisters.

This group of seven women had heard of the European doctor who could help. The doctor decided to arrive in Kampala without prior warning, thinking that this would force the issue rather than a lengthy correspondence. Professors at the University Hospital had accepted three. Another two were distributed in Christ's name to the mission hospitals, and the Belgian doctor had arrived with the two rejects at my surgeon friend's office who thence were sent to me.

Not pleased was the owner of the private hospital where I practiced, since no money could possibly change hands—and it would be a three-week stay! His charity filled him alternately with martyrdom and visions of ruin. To arrange for anesthesia and nursing for these penniless women whose smell traveled before them was a trick.

I tried to emulate Coralie Rendle-Short, my professor and fistula-repair teacher, and Professor Chassar Moir, whom I had visited in Oxford during my stay in London, specially to observe fistula repair. Professor Chassar Moir had so many students visiting that he had developed a habit of sitting on one side of the patient while operating, rather than centrally which would block the line of vision of visitors. I watched him repair a difficult post-irradiation fistula with his gentle and persuasive long fingers while a gentle rain played outside over the ancient campus. Also in my thoughts was Marion Sims, the pioneer of fistula repair in the U.S. He pitied and took into residence fistula patients and enunciated the principles of repair. Later the grateful patients became his assistants. Years later, I gazed at his statue at Central Park East and 103rd Street, the only statue commemorating a gynecologist in all of New York City.

I dissected away the bladder from the vagina, ruthlessly cut out fibrous scar tissue, and apposed the freshened bladder and vaginal edges without tension with a reconstructed wad of tissue between them.

In the days to come free and open drainage became an obsession. Golden champagne urine was happiness. A blockage caused dull panic. I often forgot these wordless women in my catheter obsession. Two weeks and some catheter training. Three weeks and the catheter out. Stay dry....stay dry.

The Belgian doctor arrived four weeks after she had entrusted her patients to my care, just as the owner of the private hospital was resigning himself to feeding these now flourishing and famished women. She collected her women from the locales where she had left them, five dry and two still leaking, already in two cruel camps: dry versus wet.

Days later I received a letter from the Belgian doctor in Butare, Rwanda. Would I like to spend a fistula week with her? She would assemble ten patients. Morning and afternoon, Monday to Friday. I had that kind of energy and had just earned freedom from breastfeeding. With much help and work flexibility, Amir and the babies would manage for a week.

On a Sunday I took a nausea-provoking flight to Kigali—Rwanda's only airport. There she was, sitting Casablanca style, on her four-wheeler parked on the runway.

There followed a hair-raising eighty miles on swervy mountain roads. Surrounding us was life in one of the world's poorest countries. Each family lived in a small hut, a clean-swept dirt yard and a *shamba* of cassava and beans. A few hens and the occasional goat. Protein-deficient red-haired children with swollen bellies lazed in the yard.

We passed a cultivated rice field, at the time the only rice in Africa. I asked the doctor about this, and she said that one afternoon there arrived at the airport a group of Chinese men and women. They came to this open space and built a small shack for themselves. The next day they went to the market and bought local implements, took them back and started clearing and cultivating the land. They planted rice and waited patiently. When the rains came and the land was flooded they replanted the shoots into the water-covered land. Before long they were harvesting the first crop. Local villagers would come and watch and learn by observation. No conversation occurred or could occur because half a world of foreignness separated them. But according to the doctor none was needed. The villagers had learned to pool their efforts, grow with only local implements, and see the results. One day, as suddenly as they came, the Chinese farmers were gone, but the fields lived on.

We arrived at her solid colonial home, with attendants waiting on our every thought. Very different at the hospital, where we went later that night to examine the two patients scheduled for the next day. The hospital beds had two heads poking out at either end. Two patients to a bed. And you had to be careful how you walked as all the beds had 'floor' patients between them.

I had been scheduled two simple soft fistulae for day one. Young women, children really, with deep age in their eyes.

Monday in the large airy cross-ventilated operating room with the windows opening onto the African countryside, quite unlike our windowless closed controlled operating rooms. I guess the fresh cross-currents of air just blew all the germs away. And natural sunlight helped the meager lighting. Soapy water from our scrubs was collected and reused to clean the sparkling floors. An easy case in the morning, home for a soporific lunch and then another in the afternoon.

Then home. The doctor lived next to green hills and we went roaming them every evening. She and, by reflected warmth, I were greeted in peasant homes with love and laughter. A woodworker presented me with a teardrop box that I still have, a weaver with an ochre and black mat.

Like the crossword puzzles in the New York Times, the cases became progressively more difficult as the week progressed. One felt as though her pelvic organs were carved out of stone. I did not have the experience, maturity or heart to reject the worst ones. I did them all.

On the Thursday evening after surgery I was waiting for my doctor friend outside the hospital. I was perched on a low stone wall, and I saw a young woman walking slowly through the opening in the stone wall that led to the front door of the hospital. She held a wad of clothing in front of her and I thought she was bringing in a sick baby. She opened the heavy double doors and disappeared from sight.

A few minutes later, the doctor appeared at the door of the hospital and called me in. The woman I saw outside was on a bed. The opened bundle lay across her abdomen. A cesarean section had been performed through a vertical skin incision ten days before and had dehisced—completely opened up. She had walked the ten odd miles to the hospital with a substantial part of her intestines wrapped in a towel. She now lay quiet with these most private of organs, pink and alive, displayed across her belly. I had a feeling of having been here before. Long years ago, through the doors of the old Women's Hospital in Bombay, a woman walked with the same stiff slow stance, the same secret load wrapped in the *palav* of her cotton sari.

We did what we had done years ago. Merciful general anesthesia, washing with floods of sterile saline to dilute out the inevitable bacteria and infection. We then returned the gone-astray contents of the abdomen back to their rightful home. We closed all in one layer with no tension on the recently ripped tissue. Antibiotics and fluids later, she miraculously recovered and said she felt well enough to go home the next day, but would stay as long as necessary.

Who are these slips of women with tenacious holds? How could she bear it? Try to enact the scene at home. For days she felt the scar stretch and become shiny thin. She covered it up and continued life in her *shamba*. I feel for her the stretch and tear as she dug and gathered, as she tended her baby, tried to breast-feed as she steamed her *matoke* and beans. She finally lay down. No one made the move to delve into what afflicted this young mother. The next morning she looked down see herself open. She saw her bowel tumbling out. Did she know what it was? Did she have someone to turn to? Anyone to take her over? Did someone bring her the rag to wrap herself in? A decision to go to the big hospital was made. Someone had to stay with the baby, so she went alone. How? Walk! Walk. Was she refused a ride once the astonishing contents of her package was seen?

My doctor friend reported complete healing and recovery. In spite of the patient's protests this time a ride was provided home.

The week flew. The doctor invited me back. An extended visit next time. Fistula time and then a trip to see the last of the world's gorillas in Virunga, the volcanic northern part of Rwanda. I meant the 'Yes' that never materialized. We parted smiling on the Kigali airstrip.

She wrote to tell me I had a 75% cure rate. How could that be? Seven and a half women cured? A dull pang identified the two or three that had to have failed. Should have desisted, been more selective.

All the 'should have' baggage one collects over the years.

Jimmy Jimereeno

When Cena was two, we started her at the same Mrs. Jones' School that Rushna had started at. Success had allowed Mrs. Jones to move from her homely garage to a spacious school building and yard just across from our home. Instead of the single class in her garage that she had started with, she now had several age-separated sections. Cena had an American teacher, Mrs. Olsen, with a twang for an accent. Come October she declared that Halloween had to be celebrated. Candy and witchy clothes were required, Cena declared. So I stitched her a 'flappy wing dress' — two squares of

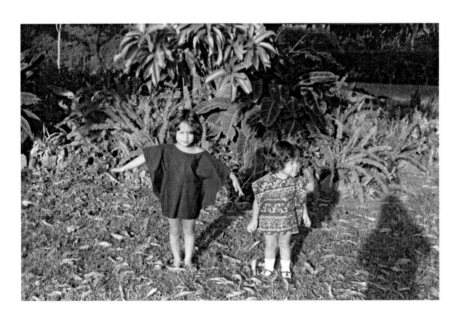

fabric stitched together at the shoulders and halfway up the sides to allow openings for the arms. I had made these all-purpose dresses for all of us out of the bright African *kitenge* fabrics, but on this occasion it was witch black.

What an enchanting brown pool-eyed curly-haired witch. She came home with masses of sweets and candy. Dentists in the U.S. must make a good living, we said to ourselves.

About a month after she had started school, Cena announced that she had a friend. 'A special friend,' she said. Jimmy, we started calling him, after J.D. Salinger's Jimmy Jimereeno. We took this calmly and with humor, till we noticed her new behavior. The food in her plate would be divided in two and one-half left uneaten. She would only occupy one-half of her bed, sit on the very edge of her chair to allow room for her friend. We watched first with amusement and then some apprehension.

Finally, I went to school to ask Mrs. Olsen who this boy was and whether Cena lived this lovelorn life at school. Mrs. Olsen told me she had not noticed anything unusual. In any case, she said, Jimmy was soon leaving this school. Relieved, I walked out and in the middle of the turmoil of playing children on the green, I saw a boy, presumably Jimmy, crouched low and two-year-old Cena standing by his side stroking his hair! I swallowed, choked, reminded myself he was leaving and walked home. Soon the sharing life she lived vanished and all was forgotten.

One day I was at a children's party and in walked Jimmy. Cena showed no sign of recognition. I pointed her friend out to her.

'Jimmy?' she asked, 'Who's he?'

1969: President of horticulture

In the 1990's Amir was a master organizer of programs for children with end-stage renal disease. He organized the first North American registry for these children, which resulted in medical management strategies that had to be accepted because of the power and strength of the studies. And he was a veritable Croesus when it came to raising money for his sick sick children. Where did he come by these skills? As I look back now, I realize he always had them.

Amir did not know a hollyhock from a ham hock, but became the president of the Uganda Horticultural Society. A few of the doctors in private practice were ardent rose and orchid cultivators. Through them he became interested, but not in the botanical aspects. He took on the raising of the funds and the organization of the annual flower show, where he did all manner of jobs from the lowliest to the grandest. I guess that was part of his magic. He managed what he had set his heart on at all levels. And he was helped by an innate generosity of spirit that always kept the big picture in sight.

At one of the flower shows he had organized, I won first prize for a floral arrangement. I cringe when I think I had any interest in this idlest of pastimes and blame it on my Parsi rearing. In a large blue and black tray-like vessel made by a local Ugandan potter, I had stood up some spectacular pink-purple ginger lilies from a corner of my 'down' garden, and then entwined long blue forget-me-not sprays through the stiff lily stems. Amir appalled the very British judges by thanking them enthusiastically and loudly, making all within hearing think my winning the prize was an arranged inside job. Whatever. This was a yearly event that people enjoyed and looked forward to. In addition to the worthless flower arrangements there were competitions for small farmers with cash prizes. And in the end, Amir always ended up in the black for the society.

Dr. C.N. Patel, a wealthy and successful local family practitioner, discovered and had an orchid named after himself—*iranga compta patelii*. He told us that this delicate small floriferous orchid that grew in great cascading bunches was to be found in the Mabira Forest on the Jinja Road. I was creating a garden heaven and the thought of growing these beauties on the mango trees would not leave my covetous heart. So one weekend, soon after the Obote shooting incident, Amir and I and the three girls drove toward Jinja and entered the Mabira Forest at a random dirt road.

Driving slowly through the lush forests, I suddenly spied a tree with branches heavy with *Iringes compta patelis*. We stopped and walked toward the tree. With Sharyn in my arms, I pointed out the branch that I coveted most. Amir walked back to the car and brought back a machete we had brought for the purpose.

Armed with this broad-bladed machete, he climbed up the tree till he got to the branch I 'needed.' He sidled onto the branch and then, before our horrified eyes, he brought the machete down on the branch between him and the tree trunk. Down came tumbling branch, Amir and all. Luckily the forest floor was as soft as a deeply padded mattress with eons of fallen vegetation and undergrowth. We untangled Amir and the prized orchids from the jumbled mess.

Amir located his machete, and just then there was a rustle in the bushes and two armed uniformed types descended on us. What could they have thought? A woman clutching onto an orchid-festooned branch in one hand and carrying a one-year-old in the other, two girls clinging onto her skirts and a disheveled bearded man brandishing a machete. Staring at Amir, they quite reasonably demanded to know what on earth we were up to. 'Orchids,' said Amir slowly and clearly, 'orchids.' Total puzzlement clouded their brows. So Amir tried another solution. 'We are doctors,' he said. '*DOCTORS*.' What that was meant to accomplish here in the jungle, I don't know, but one of the two men at once turned to him and bared his muscular midriff stating he had a pain 'right here.' Amir apologized for not having his stethoscope with him, but gave him his card and invited him to come for a free checkup and treatment anytime. Everybody was now smiling, we shook hands, they patted the children on the head and we escaped.

Everyone, but everyone, knew that the forests were being combed for Obote's attacker. Everyone except us.

The next Monday, the man came to Amir's office accompanied by wife and a brood of children. They remained his patients till we left the country.

Evolution of a cook

John Cheever, master short story writer, also known as the Ovid of Ossining, once wrote of Mary, his wife of many years whom he had long loved, used and abused. He watched her bring in the evening meal as she had done every night for more than four decades. He wrote words to this effect: 'What an achievement of depth and feeling to have nourished me daily for all these years.'

So daily cooking for the family is beyond putting food on the table. Rushna tells me one of her poignant memories was to see me come home from the hospital and go directly to the kitchen and start a meal with my raincoat still on, often glistening from the elements outside. I recall one of the few rules I had was for all of us to be at the dinner table together. Amir liked to eat late, but the children had to eat earlier or they would snack their appetites away. And there I was compromising, compromising.

I often prepared two separate meals—bland and western for the children and spicy oriental for the adults. But we, I, brought the world to the table every night. Amir expounded his extreme and powerful liberal mind...and my children never forgot that.

My earliest recollections of the way food got to the table had to do with Indian cooks, generically called *khansama*, in various military stations all over northern India. I remember the first priority of the *khansama* in Ambala—I must have been four or five—was to fill a zinc tub with water that he had heated to the boiling point in large pots over a wood fire—no running hot water. The water would be replenished through the day and used for washing dishes, for cooking and for boiling eggs—they were just tipped in as and when needed.

Later, after we settled in Bombay with my grandmother, we were fed by a master cook with a vile temperament who tolerated no interference. I realize now he was an artist who produced every variety of cuisine with flair and fervor. But he needed solitude and silence. Often he would produce things to please my grandmother's whims from pictures she showed him—a dainty filigree nougat basket filled with fruit or an aspic made in fantasy shapes. He had often neither tasted nor seen the creations he produced. His achievement was all the more wondrous because he, a Goan, ate fiery red Goa fish curry and thick-grained rice for his main two meals of the day. No question of learning anything from him.

Therefore, when I arrived in Africa, I had not the vaguest idea of how food evolved. Beset by consummate cooks in the form of Amir's mother and sisters, I was beyond out of place. I labored with cookbooks, but later learned with common sense, a good sense of taste and much advice from Ma, my mother-in-law.

She started by telling me humiliating things like, 'Remove the brown scarred end of a tomato before chopping it up,' adding, 'At least we in Africa do not eat that part.' Later I learned the principles from her. The principle of how a regular red curry evolves. The principle of going the regular spice route—tumeric, cumin, coriander, red chilli powder--or the aromatic *garam masala* route—cloves, black pepper, cinnamon, cardamom. The special way of cooking with coconut as the Swahilis do on the coast, using only garlic, lime, cilantro and green chillies so as not to overpower the coconut flavor. Once when she was watching me make *khitchri*—yellow rice with lentils—she said she would tell me a secret even Gulshan, her oldest daughter, did not know, that the flavor was improved with garlic. Such a precious secret. Since then, I have always used garlic in *khitchri* and until now I have not told this secret to anyone, not even my oldest daughter.

Once she was instructing me on how to make *moothia*, an elaborate dish with a multitude of vegetables, meat, beans, spiced dumplings made of millet flour and exotics like fenugreek. She insisted on all the ingredients being prepared separately before being assembled and would not tolerate any of my shortcuts. Eventually, after hours of fussing around slaving for her, there came the time to make the dumplings. She unceremoniously pushed me aside saying, ' Nergi, tane nahee avre,' —'Nergi, you will never be able to do this.'

There was a most delectable sweet bread—a rice-flour base with coconut milk and spices, risen with yeast. Ma would start the process at night after we had done dinner. Having mixed and loved the mixture, I saw her disappearing with it into her bedroom. Since she did not reappear, I went to investigate. She was in bed ready for sleep. She told me that the bread had to rise in a warm place and the ideal temperature was under her bed where it sagged most, giving way to her comfortable weight. This was not a recipe I would use.

Her method of measuring pleased me, and to everyone's exasperation, I still use it. When asked how much of an ingredient was to be used, she would oppose her thumb to her four fingers. If it was a little, she would put her thumb near her fingertips, further down if it was more, and so on.

And then there was an array of birthday cakes.

I have just returned from Washington, D.C. It is election day, 2004—the most important election of our lifetime. But however it turns out, I am refreshed by my grandson Kiran's birthday, especially by the creation of a cake made to order. He said he needed two mountains, one with a tunnel and an active volcano, with twin tracks, and one for a train and one for racecars running over and through the scenery. 'No problem,' said mother Sharyn. Two (cake mix—shame) mounds, one gouged out with a tunnel iced garishly. A bundt for the volcano—filled with bright red molten icing in danger of exploding at any moment. Licorice railroad tracks and Hershey chocolate squares for car tracks and plentiful railroad and car props. All was displayed on a giant foil-lined cardboard square.

Wild birthday cakes may not seem like much, but I have given this to my children. From the time they were little, they ordered and I created: pussycats—two unequal rounds with the cutout parts forming tail and ears; Barbie dolls—a giant dome decorated as a skirt with a real Barbie doll messily plunged in up to her waist; a butterfly—four rounds, two large and two small—with cut-outs forming the body and feelers, an improvement on any real butterfly; a house made of a loaf cake iced and slope-roofed in graham crackers with a garden filled with improbable flowers, all smothered in icing and fanciful candy. And so they continue. Cena, who demanded the most fanciful cakes, now has rejected this nonsense and has good-tasting conventional layer cakes—though she did insist on a Taj Mahal cake for her wedding.

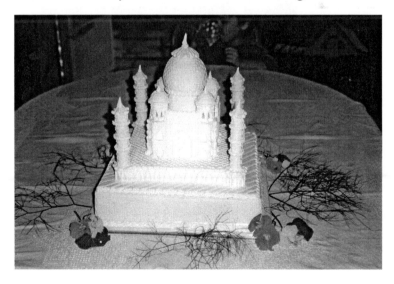

But the rest have had dinosaurs, trains, cars, volcanos. Ellis, my oldest grandson, announced his maturity on his twelfth birthday by saying that if his mother had to make a cake, a round one would suffice.

Bella and Len

Through Aneel Korde, now married to Amir's sister Laila, we got to know Jonathan and Elena Kingdon. Jonathan was an artist and taught at the School of Fine Arts at Makerere University. He was born in Tanzania and was quite unlike a transplanted Caucasian born in England—easy, laughing and open. Or maybe it was just him. Elena was Italian and thoroughly nice, but seemed to have an undercurrent of uneasiness that contrasted with his fine comfort. They had children with grand African names. One of them, Fofu (fish), was Cena's age, and they would have frequent play dates. One afternoon when Cena was with the Kingdons, Jonathan made a pencil sketch of her. I have this likeness in my living room. It

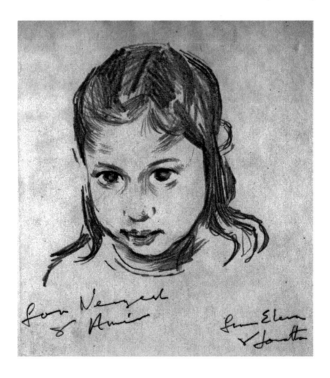

captured perfectly that lovely heart-shaped face, eyes like pools and lips that were full and never needed any assistance as they were bright pink. One day I will give it to Cena, now a doctor, but presently I still need it for my pleasure.

On one occasion we were invited to dinner at the Kingdons and seated at the table were Bella and Len Feldman. Len was a mathematician on a two-year grant from Columbia University to develop a math curriculum for Ugandan high schools. Bella was a sculptor who became a faculty member in the School of Fine Arts with Jonathan. They had lived their early years in New York and later left the steel and glass temples for the open spaces of Berkeley, California.

The talk turned to the American involvement in Vietnam. Amir—who I could see was totally taken by Bella's intelligence, beauty, wit and ability to roll off four-letter words with ease and aplomb and absolutely no self-consciousness—baited her, making her out to be representative of the great clumsy powerful U.S. behemoth. He was properly put in his place when she and Len described their involvement in the protest movement and their eventual disgust, which caused them to leave and take this position in Uganda.

Bella called the next day to come to our home, ostensibly to borrow a book we had talked of the night before, but actually to open the door to a friendship that has lasted over time, distances and the death of both our male partners. I saw her a few nights ago, lovely and peaceful with a new gentle love—but still protesting.

Her latest exhibition, 'War Toys,' inspired by and against the U.S. involvement in Iraq, has not been well received because of the mood in this country.

Bella and Len invited us to participate in their observation of the Seder that year. While the feast was traditional, the ambience was revolutionary. Danny, their young curly-haired son, asked the questions. And what questions! Instead of 'Why is this night like no other night?' the questions were pointed and directed toward the illegal, brutal war being fought against an innocent people many thousands of miles from the shores of the U.S. Bella later told me that not everyone was as impressed as we were. There were some traditionalists at the table who thought this was a desecration of an ancient rite and sacred night.

But to us it was seductive. Besides the protest in its literal sense, there was something else. We were living in a country which was rapidly turning into a one-party state with an all-powerful leader. Our Asian race was being marginalized and ostracized, and there was no question of protest, for fear of reprisal. To be able to express opposition freely was new and resuscitating to us. We told of and remembered that Seder night many, many times.

We had many other pleasure-filled times together. In their second year they talked to us about our future in this country. We were still blinded by our being Ugandan and thought it paranoiac to anticipate disaster. Bella said something which we never forgot: 'Only the paranoiac Jews lived to tell their tale.'

In 1970, after we had made the decision to emigrate to the U.S., the Feldmans helped us to move our small savings to the U.S. Len was paid in the U.S. and deposited funds in an account in our name in the U.S., and we paid them the equivalent in Uganda. Sounds fishy, but it worked. People asked what interest they charged. The answer—only in friendship. The money the Feldmans helped us with became the down payment on our first home in the U.S., in Garden City, New York, a ranch-style house with the living and dining rooms forming an 'L.' Just like the lovely Roscoe Road house we had left behind.

SEVEN

Leaving Uganda

1970: Preparations to go West

For my children there are two things in my life I wish I could find words to describe in their entire truth. First, the entire lack of any traditional form of religion. And second, the impetus, urge and deed to leave the country of one's birth and move. Forever looking for something. Religion some other time.

I had a distant relative from my old home in Bombay who visited me in Kampala. His name was LL—a mild and lovely man with a wife as unlike him as ever could be possible—acidic, doomful, complete with witch's wart and cutting tongue. But he was softly shapeless, softly spoken and soft, so soft. He lived all his life in Bombay in an old apartment at Grant Road from birth to his retirement and eventually to his death. He worked as a pillar of non-corruption in the Bank of India in the city. Every morning of his working life he took the 9.15 a.m. commuter train to Churchgate Station and was back to his unlovely wife on the 6 p.m. Once a month he would satisfy his lust for Western classical music and go to the Cowasji Jehangir Hall for a concert by the Bombay Philharmonic or a visiting orchestra. He went alone as his wife had no taste for this. His visit to Kampala was quiet and pleasant as he spoke to me of my father's father, Manekji Bharucha, a city planner and theosophist whom I never knew. LL was a tree rooted forever to the place of his birth, content in spite of wife and childlessness. And it was not for lack of the adventurous spirit, for he had climbed and knew the heights of great music and world literature, all in the comfort of his armchair.

I had migrated before we left for America. Sometimes I think of it like a man-eating tiger, who, though old and with powerful teeth weakened, had once tasted human blood and now had to do it again. And Amir's father had migrated. Whatever your parents had done seemed okay to do again. We never stayed anywhere long enough for roots to appear. And yet today I see distinct and strong roots evident in my children. My grandchildren are completely rooted in this U.S.A.

The reasons for migration are diverse, but I can only muse upon those that were close to me in the restless Asian community in Uganda. Most small Indian businesspeople in Uganda had an undying loyalty and pledge to India. The minority of these were primary immigrants—most were born in East Africa. Many had never been to India, and yet the tie was tight and forever. I read in Gareth Barberton's memoirs of his pride as an Englishman, in spite of his Kenyan birth and difficulties of establishing British citizenship. This must be a primitive and original emotion alien to me.

This bond to India was in very large part responsible for the dangerous situation of the Indians in East Africa. Most maintained Indian citizenship. Some families established Ugandan citizenship for some family members to 'look good.' Most had a piece of land in *desh*—back home. They eventually gathered the money to build a house in readiness for retirement in the home of their hearts. And how did it look from the outside? That they milked Africa for a living while creating a far-away home of the heart. Uganda was a temporary stop for most. No matter that my immediate and Amir's extended family were Ugandan, no matter that we had no possessions outside Uganda and no matter that we had no home outside Uganda—we were massed with all people of our color.

Destinations for emigration by the East African Asian community were dictated by religious and by economic considerations. The India thing represented the feelings of the Hindu small businesspersons. The more affluent Hindus, the Ismailis and the minute Parsi community looked to the West. They, too, regarded themselves as only in transit. Many had British passports, blatantly stamped 'D,' as opposed to the regular passports of regular Britishers. 'D' for devalued, they ruefully or angrily declared. Yet despite the racially charged British policies, they thought to eventually enter Britain, even making provisions for this eventuality. Others directed themselves to the more hospitable Canada—a substantial community now resides in Vancouver, British Columbia.

And then there were a few, like us, who had no thought of leaving till the end of 1969. By this time, the Obote autocracy, with the help of army strongman Idi Amin, was established. Opposition parties were decimated. Many adults had never voted. The newspapers were mouthpieces of the party, and each day the papers contained some real or imagined Asian act of disloyalty. Rushna, aged six, was an outstanding student and already showed the speed-reading talent that was and is among her finest possessions. The nursery and elementary schools were fine, but deterioration loomed at higher levels. Friends, foremost Len and Bella, gave us warning of impending catastrophe.

As soon as the doubts started, we were restless. Determined not to go back to the land of our ex-masters nor to Canada, where many were headed, we set our minds, if not our hearts, on the United States, a land created on the philosophy of the riches of the immigrant—'....not merely a nation but a teeming nation of nations.' Once we started the process, it was quite painless. Few Asians were directed there, and there was quick efficient service and short lines. Unlike what happened later, there was a need for doctors and vacancies at resident levels because of young doctors being drafted into the Viet Nam conflict. Because of our previous experience, I was required to do only two years of a four-year residency in Ob/Gyn, and Amir needed only two of a standard three-year pediatric residency. We looked into positions in proximity to each other. The first positive reply came from Tulane in the American South. How different life would have been if this had materialized. But they soon wrote and said that for reasons I cannot remember, my position would be of observer only! So we persisted and obtained resident positions in Brooklyn. My third-year resident position at the Methodist Hospital of Brooklyn had been created when the incumbent was drafted to Viet Nam. The Chairman, Dr. Clemetson, a Britisher, recognized my MRCOG degree and favored me over other applicants. Amir got a second-year position at the Brooklyn Jewish Hospital.

Bella gave us a detailed city planner-type map of Brooklyn, and we pored over our future. The map showed a jungle of apartment buildings and complicated city streets. But I did see with relief the big green Prospect Park, the public library, the Brooklyn Botanical Gardens and the Brooklyn Museum all gathered around a heroic monument, the Grand Army Plaza...all seemingly in walking distance from the Methodist Hospital and resident quarters where we were assigned a two-bedroom apartment on the third floor. We were to spend the first two years of our life in the U.S. in Brooklyn, and thirty years later Cena and her little family were to live a few blocks away from our first home. And I now visit there once a week, to show Cena's daughter Tehmina the trees her mother climbed, the rocks in the garden where she picnicked, the playground where she did her nimble handstands.

The positions were contingent upon our passing a qualifying examination, the Educational Council for Foreign Medical Graduates (ECFMG), which was given every three months in Kampala. When Amir said he was registering us to appear, I arrogantly told him to appear first, and if and when he passed, I guaranteed I would pass three months later. He often told this tale as evidence of my arrogance and rudeness. He did pass, and so I had to. The test was in all clinical specialties, so some reading had to be done. But the hardest part was the English test, where one had to make sense of the nasal twang that the reader of the text claimed was English. She read some inane passage and we had to answer questions on it to illustrate comprehension. Close attention allowed me to hear, if not understand, something about her aunt coming home for Thanksgiving—a holiday I had never heard of, but years later took to my heart.

The process of leaving was now inevitable. I kept looking at familiar things and looking again, for it was a last time. The water lilies, the *mohur* on the mango trees our wild orchid *Iringa compta patelis* now cascading from the mango trees. The stone slabs we played on. Goodbye, male and female papayas. The long lovely living room. The blond Elgon olive-wood furniture. The democratic round dining table.

We sold our house to Mr. Kataramu, whose later murder at our doorstep I have recounted. He bought the house with its furniture, our crockery, cutlery, kitchen utensils, our stereo, even the books we left behind. He paid us in cash, which he brought in a small suitcase, which we got out of the country, but I cannot recall how. A Swiss bank whose code number I have misplaced was involved.

We were to leave at the end of June of 1971. Suddenly misgivings plagued me. To face this whole 'of another color,' speaking with a different accent yet again, convinced me we must have a masochistic streak, further substantiated by the certain knowledge that the ECFMG was only an entry test for the U.S. Later would come the licensing exams, the specialty board exams and the subspecialty tests that we would both take. None of this would have been required in England, Canada or India.

I convinced Amir that we should pay a last visit to India before our departure. I always notice, even now, a certain loss of tension as soon as I land in India--loss of a tension I didn't even know I possessed, the relaxation caused by a brown person dissolving into the brown masses. Let's look and see if there is a chance for us back in that ancient land. He agreed and we arranged to go. It was the children's first time in India, in March of 1971. But in January of that year a major upheaval occurred in that lovely green land we were leaving.

1971: The coup

On the morning of January 25th, 1971, Amir's father called us and said there was something afoot. He did not know what it was, but asked us and the children to stay home from work and school. We switched on the radio, and instead of the usual pro-government anti-Asian banalities there was the blandest of music. 'In the shade of an old apple tree' still brings back that troubled day. It was an army-band non-vocal rendition. A more unsuited ditty for that occasion I cannot imagine.

'In the shade of the old apple tree,
Where the love in your eyes I can see,
With a heart that is true I'll be waiting for you,
In the shade of the old apple tree.'
There were no apple trees in Uganda.
This played chillingly through the day.

Every time it ended we waited, but its bland tones just started again.

And then, at about three in the afternoon, it stopped. An unknown announcer in impeccable BBC English announced General Idi Amin, later to assume exalted self-endowed titles, all of which ended in 'for life.'

He addressed us in English, heavily accented from the north where he was born, perhaps not even in Uganda but across the border in Sudan. Like the wild and magnificent wildebeeste, zebra and deer who migrate across boundaries in search of rain, he had recognized no boundary and drifted into Uganda. It started as a humble-soldier speech, recounting the sins of Obote's autocratic ways, all true. He vowed to retire to his barracks, like the soldier that he was, as soon as stability was restored and a civilian government put in place. He then addressed the minorities—me and mine—and assured us that if we 'parcipitated' in working toward the good of our Uganda, we would have nothing to fear. Always after, when Amir or I used the word, we said, 'parcipitate.'

He had taken this moment to claim Uganda, as Obote was at a Commonwealth Conference in Singapore. Later, we knew that Obote had resolved to oust Amin, who had become too strong and independent, when he returned. Amin was making a pre-emptive strike.

Even as he spoke we heard the joyous crowds taking to the streets on Kampala Road. We went out to see the jubilation and wondered if we were making a wrong turn in leaving this now-promising situation.

Before long the crowds gathered on Kampala Road were frenzied to see Amin in khakis, unprotected and unafraid, through the throng, driving his own jeep. A sharp contrast to Obote who had taken to armored cars and bullet-proof vests. He stopped, laughed, waved and slowly drove off.

We had no idea, but the killings had already started—killings that were soon to choke the Nile with human bodies they hoped the crocodiles would look after.

Amin at the pool

We were still planning on looking over India before making our move. But while in Uganda, we maintained our usual activities. One was a weekend swim at the pool at the Apollo Hotel, named after Apollo Milton Obote, the now ousted President.

We initially went to the Silver Springs Pool, some miles out of Kampala. This was a traditional rectangular pool in leafy green surroundings. I taught Rushna, a quick learner with no fear of the water, to swim in this pool. When the Apollo Pool was built, we started using it because it was closer and grander. It was round and Disneyesque, a bright unbelievable shade of blue, complete with a central island, bridge and staged water cascades. I have always hated round pools as both pretentious and impossible to swim laps in. Swimming interminably around the pool was tiring and caused an asymmetry of stroke, exercising one-half of the body differently from the other. But we loved the ambience, and I taught Cena and Sharyn to swim in this pool. Cena learnt quietly and swiftly. But Sharyn displayed her life-long habit of incessant chatter when nervous. In spite of swallowed, inhaled, and coughed water, she kept up her nervous prattle till she got the hang of it. She now speeds ahead of me in an elegant crawl.

In February, one of these last weekends at the Apollo Pool, we turned toward the direction where people were craning. Walking into the pool area was Idi Amin, assorted women and several children. Only when seen at close quarters did one realize the charisma of the man. Huge, ebon and shining with a constant laugh.

His children all jumped into the pool with much splashing and laughter. All except one skinny little six or seven-year-old, who clung to his mother's skirts. Amin walked over to the child and boomed encouragement to jump in. The child clung closer to his mother. This mountainous man then lifted the screaming child high in the air, walked to the pool edge and flung him in.

All eyes were on Amin, still grotesquely smiling, and the near-drowning child. As long as Amin stood there, no one dared to rescue the child. Then some trace of humanity must have moved him, and he turned his back on the boy, inviting rescue. As soon as his back was turned, someone jumped in and brought the child out to his mother. Both left the pool area hurriedly.

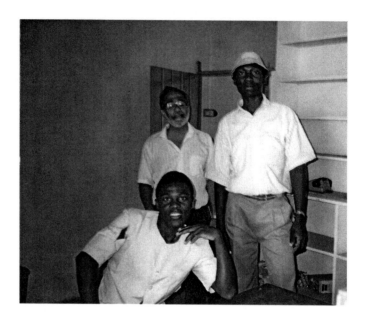

Unfinished business

How does one end eleven years in Africa? For Amir, it was a lifetime with many wandering years away while studying. And for my children, it was all their lives.

Our house was already sold to Mr. Kataramu. We tried to sell our practices, but had no buyers. So since both offices were rented, we just gave away the furnishings and few surgical instruments and did not renew our leases. Years later, when we went back in 1992, Amir's office was a bar with three jolly young men running it. We stopped, had a drink with them and took pictures.

We managed to secure jobs for Elena, the ayah, and Leopold, the Congolese gardener. We got a job for Ramzani as well, but months later, while in the U.S. we heard that his new employer was very upset because he continued to do what he had always done with us--help himself to flour, oil, sugar, rice. I did not see the problem with it. But the new regime saw it differently.

We planned a visit to India in March with the thought of visiting my sisters before plunging deeper into the West and to take a last look at whether we could make a life as brown people in a brown country.

A last look at India

In March of 1971 we flew to Bombay on a United Arab Airways (UAA) flight. With all the flying we had to do, we did not want to deplete our small savings. And UAA undercut all other airlines. One could even bargain with them—which Amir felt right at home doing. It was a time when several hijackings had occurred and people asked us if we were not apprehensive of this. To which Amir replied, 'We are perfectly safe because we are flying with the hijackers' airline.'

All UAA flights converged on Cairo and then there was a free-for-all to get our connection, during which there was always time to visit that astounding city. A camel ride at the Giza pyramids. And then we climbed to the top of the ancient pyramid in a claustrophobic chute leading to a disappointing small chamber with, as far as I remember, nothing in it. My children and I stared and stared at the Sphinx. She told us nothing. Come on, Sphinx, are we making a happy move? No answer.

Later we went to an ornate sateen-tented perfume palace. All the perfumes of Arabia in thousands of glass and crystal containers glinted and squinted at us. Rose attar straight from the cabbage roses in my round garden. The mysterious Arab demonstrating the perfumes rubbed a smidgeon of each perfume and oil on to the back of my hand and then endearingly into the children's hair. He tried Amir's hand but recoiled at the stare he got. My children and I swayed out intoxicated. Amir who theoretically regarded Arabs as his brothers, suspected every move an Arab made around his female coterie.

After several false alarms we finally boarded our connection to Bombay. I tried to prepare my children for their first visit to where their mother was born. Where I met their father. Where he and I walked everywhere in a love haze. Where we were married.

But you can never prepare for your first visit to Bombay. It started with an orderly line at the customs desk. The single customs officer strolled in yawning about half an hour after the line formed. He started work after he adjusted his ragged chair, cleared his throat with a resounding blood-curdling hawk and a really satisfying stream of red-tinged, betel-nut heavy spittle, after he had cleaned his glasses on a rag that appeared to have previously been used on the underbelly of an oily car. And, of course, after a scurrying underling had brought him a milky cup of steaming tea, which he poured into the saucer to cool and then slurped with gusto. As soon as he took his place the orderly line changed into a raging mob which my girls and I shrank from. But Amir (I suddenly realized one of the reasons I had married him) had a briefcase in his hand and, using it as a weapon, forged a path through the roiling seas and before we knew it we were with my waiting sister, Shirin.

I had not seen Shirin since our father had died. Meeting the first time after a mutual loss is full of injury, and we tried to balance ourselves. Amir was the leavening agent, and we survived. But then that drive from the airport to 'Court View,' my old and now Shirin's home, through Dharavi, the worst slum in the world. Thousands of people displaced from the villages, scratching a living from the big city. Generations had lived and continue to live there. A single water source. No sewage system—lines of humanity squatting to defecate on the nearby railroad tracks with a *lota*—a brass container—of water to wash. Hovels too low to accommodate a standing person, built of sticks, sackcloth, newspaper and plastic with the more fortunate using strips of corrugated metal—all washed away and refurbished with each ferocious monsoon season. How could I prepare anyone, much less my tender children, for this?

Mercifully, they slept through the ride—the time was two in the morning. At 'Court View,' there were pavement-dwellers we had to step over to get to the familiar old wood-lined elevator with pastoral scenes of different hued woods, a genuine old Wrigley which predated Otis elevators. Up to the fourth floor to be greeted by Cecilia, Shirin's maid of all jobs and chef extraordinaire. She had readied the entry ceremony, which Shirin performed. This time it was from the book because it was the first for my girls.

The five of us stood just outside the heavy wooden door, whose transom was garlanded. On the floor were colored chalk stencils of symmetrical design and lucky fish shapes. On a silver tray were the ornate containers for the red *kum-kum*, a rose-water shaker, and a funnel (dunce-cap) with a garland of roses twisted around it, filled with rock sugar. Also on the tray were acquisitions from Hindu culture, a perfectly heart-shaped betel-nut leaf and a betel nut. A good-luck silver flexible fish with ruby eyes. A few dried dates and a dried coconut signifying the desert of our Persian ancestors and a silver bowl of uncooked rice. We were garlanded in roses and tuberoses, the coconut was circled over our heads to ward away the evil eye and, to my children's delight, crashed against the sturdy floor to split it open. A red dot was placed on our foreheads, a piece of rock sugar on our tongues and rice pressed into the forehead red dot and scattered over us. We entered the house right foot first for good luck. My children had started to enjoy this lovely attention. A few hours of rest and we were ready to go.

The next morning I led them slowly through the apartment, telling of the good things that had happened there. I left out the bad things. The terrazzo-tiled multi-colored floor in the living room had a perfect hopscotch plan—impossible as far as décor, but perfect for restless children. And then secret bookcases, now unlocked, with old books. Old photographs of the grandparents and great grandparents they would never meet. Old China and silverware, for which I have a nostalgia but no desire.

We sat down to a celebratory Parsi breakfast on a shining white damask cloth spread over the old polished oversized dining table. Homemade yogurt made of buffalo milk, so creamy and thick it could cut like a cake. Cream of wheat, not the instant stuff, but made from gallons of milk boiled down to a toffee thickness, decorated with cardamom, nutmeg, toasted almonds and raisins and, Sharyn's favorite, pink rose petals. Spicy fried pomfret fish and then, to add a light touch, hard-boiled eggs. Rushna and Cena were a Jack Spratt act. Rushna always ate the yellow and Cena the white of the egg. Between the two they 'licked the platter clean.'

A typical city-dweller, Shirin had no car but a friend lent us one for the day, complete with chauffeur, and we went on a tour of this island city, previously several islands, now joined with reclaimed land, which had been given as a dowry by the King of Portugal to the English monarch Charles II when he married the Portuguese princess Catherine of Braganza in 1662.

Spring was the time of the 'Holi' festival when people don their oldest clothes and take to the streets to joyfully, mischievously and sometimes malignantly spray water-based paints on each other. The way one sees politicians in the West lighting Christmas trees and serving turkey to show they are one with the common folk, there would be yearly photographs of creaky old male and some female politicians with studied smiles reluctantly spraying paint on each other's clothes. I remember a long-ago picture of that noble-faced Nehru, who seemed to be genuinely enjoying himself, frolicking with his daughter Indira on Holi day.

Hot pink, peacock blue and aqua-soaked urchins surrounded our car at a traffic intersection. They opened the car door and sprayed us all. A harmless rite that somehow did not sit well. The 'have-nots' reduced the chauffeur-driven, English-speaking 'haves' to their level. The children did not laugh, and I realized I had to present this India in small vetted doses.

We tried to stay by the ocean, which always looks magnificent. We walked on Marine Drive, a main promenade close to our home. And though the facing row of apartment buildings was in disrepair because of weathering the serious south-west monsoon winds and rain each year, there was something friendly and communal on the promenade. No such central gathering place existed in Kampala.

We stopped for coconuts and watched as the tops were sliced thin with murderous sharp knives and then uncapped to access the water. At the roasted peanuts and chickpea sellers, a few paisas bought us a crunchy hot snack. We passed a gate leading to the rocks by the sea, where a group of Parsis were praying the sea prayer and retying their sacred thread, the *kasti,* over their fine *sadra* undershirt—finest cotton, or more modern net with lace lining—all the while intoning the *Kemna Mazda* prayer to seal the knots in the thread with good thoughts, good words and good deeds.

More impressively further down near the Hindu area there was a *sadhu,* stark naked and ash covered, and several yogis doing their constitutional headstands. Then there were the regular masses— masses and masses of people, some in sneakers and shorts walking determinedly, some jogging, some ambling, some ogling. Quiet couples held hands. And then the jasmine sellers. Years before Amir would never pass them without getting a jasmine bracelet for my wrist. We got them for the children and the smell made us all relax.

Crawford Market was another lovely place. By now the children were learning to look above street level, seeing this new place with their new eyes. The cavernous hall to the right of the entrance

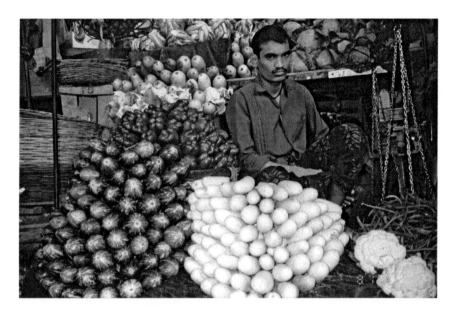

was the flower market. Little stalls decorated with sweetest roses, tuberoses, marigolds and gladioli. And then a whole row of stalls with grown men busily weaving jasmine and marigold into single, double and triple-strand bracelets and garlands. A flower and a surgeon's knot, another and another. Beautiful square knots that never came undone and were discarded intact when the flowers died the next day. It is an infectious custom, and we had jasmine bracelets every day.

Straight ahead were the vegetable markets with each little stall arranged like a Cezanne still life. Pyramids of reddest tomatoes, circles of white and purple eggplants. Bunches and bunches of radish, scallions and carrots. And the greens of coriander, fenugreek, dill and wide-leaved spinach—so much water on their fresh leaves that shaking them out soaked us. We decided against taking the children to the fish-market hall. And we certainly were not going to the Ballard pier, where the fishermen and women first brought in the fish. Fish of every sort were piled high on the sidewalks with stray dogs walking and helping themselves freely to the piles. Fisherwomen dressed in the tight seductive Maharashtrian nine-yard sari (the usual sari is six yards) tightly draped between the legs to give a pants-type freedom. These women screamed at customers, bargained until only anger ended the deal, and on occasion threw dead fish at people who displeased them or in good humor to seal a bawdy joke.

A few days in Bombay were enough, and we took the long train ride to Mathura, the ancient religious capital of India, and were greeted at the station by Perrin, my older sister. Her husband, Jehangir Sataravala, a general in the Indian Army, was the army commander based at Mathura. We drove through the crowded streets to the cantonment area, to their spacious house teeming with aides, gardeners, cooks and other indeterminates. My children met their cousins, Perrin's children, Shekufay, Tina, Cyrus and Jehan. They had met Shekufay previously when she had visited us in Kampala, but the rest were a first time. It was a happy meeting, Perrin's children in their fluent but North-Indian-accented English and mine in British-tinged English.

The General would work in the mornings and end his day at about two in the afternoon. He would come in his general's regalia and sit in his special chair. A man would come scurrying in and loosen the laces of his mirror-shining shoes and help ease them off. Cena watched this ritual round-eyed every day and finally declared to her sisters, 'Poor man does not know how to undo his own shoelaces.'

Behind the general's house flowed the Yamuna River on its way to meet the Ganga at the sacred *sangam* in Allahabad before the united rivers flowed on to the Bay of Bengal. Evenings we would walk by the Yamuna while Jehangir would tell tales of old battles and bygone family adventures.

Once we passed a man squatting by and staring into the river, and Perrin told us the story of the melon growers. These folk lived in their makeshift huts by the Yamuna. In the dry season, which should have been at this time, they would plant melon seeds in the fertile dried riverbeds. The melons would grow fast and furiously. Selling them would provide income for the rest of the year and sustain them and their families while the river flowed till next year's dry season. This year the river did not dry up, and the melon growers were left with no farmland. The man sitting by the river was an idle melon grower. Knowing of his tragedy, as we passed, Perrin asked him in Hindi, 'What will you do this year?' This man, who had no material possession one could discern, said with no anger, 'Nadi deti hai, nadi leti hai.' 'The river gives and the river takes.'

The children were royalty, and Jehangir had their sausages and bacon brought in daily in a special order from Delhi on the mail train.

An air-conditioned train ride to Agra took us to the moonlit Taj Mahal. Surrounding the monument, people were selling inlay work like the panels on the Taj. They used simple manually run grinding wheels to shape the marble petals for inlay. And I could see them inhaling marble dust day after day as no doubt Shah Jehan's artisans had done centuries ago when he built that monument to his dead love, Mumtaz Mahal. Does this help when your beloved has gone? Building a vast magnificent edifice, putting thousands to work for a monument to your love, seeing the whole city directed toward your queen. Instead of the world going its way and people returning to their business, leaving you with your empty bed.

For added flourish, the story goes, at the completion of the Taj Mahal, he had the artisans' hands cut off so they could never repeat this design. For all his sins, his son imprisoned him in an edifice further up the river which faced away from the Taj so that he could never see it. But an artfully placed mirror tile, put in by a faithful worker, reflected the Taj in miniature.

Less well known, but also in Agra, is the more contemporary Birla Temple. I remembered its beauty from a visit while a medical student. Because of the intricacy of the sculpture, it was decades in the making, with generations of family artisans involved. The temple was a paean to the garden. Curving cucumber vines, cascading tomato plants, eggplant sentinels, beans showering from the transoms. We were all delighted and as far as we knew no hands were chopped off to retain its uniqueness.

On our return to Mathura, Perrin took me and the girls to the Mathura Market. Amir wisely decided to stay home in the luxury of the khus-khus-cooled house—great absorbent drenched grass screens at each door—that were moved back and forth by a person, often a child, to keep the interior of the house cool. Iced beer and any amenity one desired brought on a silver salver added to the attraction of staying home.

We were driven to the Mathura Market in a staff car which

had to stop before the pedestrians-only market. We disembarked to the embarrassing stiff salute of the driver and followed Perrin in her *chappals* and cotton sari, picking her way easily through street vendors, goats, cows, touts, and ash-covered *sadhus*. Our destination was the *chitalwalla*—the glass bangle seller. Before we got to him, we stepped over every form of human and human refuse imaginable.

Unforgettably, we passed a man sitting on the dirt selling sweets, white *barfi*, saffron red *jalebi*, pistachio green something else. He sat immobile, covered with flies on all the exposed parts of his body with no sign of annoyance or effort to remove them. I have often thought of that man. Can one tolerate extreme poverty better if one is non-reactive? Was it so hopeless a task because the sweets were a constant attraction to flies? Was it more practical, in that the more flies on him, the fewer on the sweets? In the end, I remember it as an act of total faith in what was to be and the inability to change destiny.

The *chitalwalla*'s roadside store was a joy. Hundreds, maybe thousands of glass bangles on rods balanced every which way, but beautifully color-coordinated. For greater effect, the man, a wisp of a person, put alternative color combinations on his own fragile wrists and swayed his hands in a snake-like motion. No million-dollar model could have been more enticing, and the children were enchanted, making him break into wilder motion. We bought a dozen of every color you can think of and some colors you could not. Glass bangles break with a frequency that makes them a disposable item. For reasons difficult to explain, they never cause injury even when they break on your wrist.

On our return, I had a headache, very unusual for me, and Perrin said she had the perfect remedy. She instructed a messenger who sped off as he was told. About half an hour later, a man who had to be more than a hundred years old, fragile and weighing no more than eighty pounds with a severe tremor, walked in armed with bottles of oils. Under Perrin's guidance we were taken to the bathroom where the ancient proceeded to climb into the bathtub. I had no idea of what was expected of me. A communal bath? No, I was told, sit on the stool by the side of the bathtub with your back to him. It was further explained that when he performed, he tended to lose his balance and being in the bathtub stabilized him. He then applied oils selected for my ailment (pounding frontal headache) and started a vibratory massage that had to be experienced to be believed. As he went into a frenzy of vibrations, he would gradually keel to one or the other side, and Perrin standing by would shove him back to the upright position. This went on unabated for thirty minutes. His performance made me completely forget about my headache.

After this, cool water was brought for him and, thus revived, he nimbly jumped out of the bathtub and thanked me for the privilege of massaging my head. After he had accepted some money while fiercely protesting, Perrin's son Cyrus asked him for a haircut. He was a man of many talents. From his dingy pocket came out scissors and razors, and with tremulous hands he gave Cyrus a smart haircut, drawing blood only once. To cut the general's son's hair was such an honor that he flatly refused payment. Perrin later paid him in kind—a meal and some clothing for his womenfolk.

Our plan was to spend a few days in Delhi and Kashmir and then leave the children with Perrin in Mathura so we could go to the U.S. and smooth the way before we made our final exit. Perrin was to bring the children to Cairo, the great meeting place for all UAA flights, and then would come back to Kampala with us for a holiday and to help pack up our lives.

We toured Luyten's New Delhi, one of the few planned cities of the world, with symmetry and pomp and circumstance in every corner. Decades later I was in Pretoria and had a flush of déjà vu. A transparency of New Delhi over Pretoria would fit exactly. Luytens had been here, too. Who was this man who traveled continents designing sterile empty capital cities?

Old Delhi was stifling but held extreme beauty. The Red Fort, from which Indian prime ministers make their yearly Independence Day speech, is a marvel. Adding to the vista are the sari dyers outside the Fort who tint six yards of sari with vivid hues and hold them up to flap in the torrid wind.

We saw a sound and light show at the Fort with a recreation of life in Mughal times. Tittering women, playing fountains. Baths of every shape in marble and stone—all enveloped in the whispering shadowed imageless lattice work of Islam.

Not completely forgetting the purpose of our visit, we arranged to meet a physician at the All India Institute of Medicine, the premier medical school and research institute of the country. Nothing worked out at this assignation. The physician we were to meet was late, and we wandered the gloomy corridors of the hospital with large general wards and floor patients. When the doctor finally came, he was so harassed and beset by clinical problems that it was impossible to engage him in anything meaningful. We did learn that the salary would be impossible and we would each have to work at least one other full-time job to anywhere near making ends meet. Four full-time jobs between the two of us was not appealing. We set the India thoughts away forever.

A short flight took us to Srinagar in Kashmir. Fifty years of violent tussle over this beauteous land has decimated it, but we visited while it was still the garden it had been in the time of the Mughal kings. In the taxi from the airport to Dal Lake, Amir asked the driver why they would not settle for Indian rule after all the money and beneficence India had poured into Kashmir. He asked the question fully knowing the answer from this Moslem amongst Moslems. The taxi driver answered that it was true that India had helped Kashmir, but, said he, when he died only his Moslem brethren would 'give a shoulder to his coffin.' Amir often described to me the deep significance attached to this last rite, where male family and friends put their shoulders to the coffin and move seamlessly in relays so that as many as possible have touched their shoulders to the dead.

We spent a few enchanted days on a houseboat on Dal Lake with Perrin's daughters, Shekufay and Tina. Early morning, the *shikaras*, small decorated rowboats with fanciful names, would come to our houseboat to sell their wares. Loveliest of all was the flower-seller with the small boat overflowing with tulips and daffodils, flowers of temperate lands in this much-fought-over sad vale.

We rode small ponies in the wild flower-covered valleys of Khilanmarg and Gulmarg. We waded in the Jhelum River, white and bright crystal green, rushing, turbulent and freezing pure, fresh from its Himalayan source. And we always returned to our cozy houseboat to eat warm tasty meals prepared by green-eyed

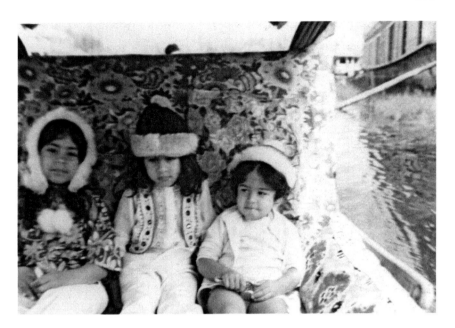

and quiet Kashmiri attendants and sleep on soft sinking beds. We were there on April 12th when Cena turned five, and we took a celebratory *shikara* ride around the lake, she, dressed in a Kashmiri cap, fine white cotton trousers and an embroidered shirt.

The boat ride reminded us of the poverty in the valley. Lovely green-eyed children, no thought of school, helping their mothers to wash clothes in the lake, carry water to their jerry-built boats. Men carrying *sigries*—charcoal stoves—hugged to their bellies to keep warm, a common cause of skin cancer because of the constant proximity to carcinogens.

We forget the poor quickly. How can one keep all of it? We'll think of it tomorrow.

The Shalimar Gardens were the ultimate in formality with every blade of grass and flower petal grown in ultimate symmetry. The Mughal Emperor Shah Jehan, who designed and created these gardens in 1632, wrote, 'If there is heaven on earth, it is this, it is this, it is this.' Heaven torn apart by a peace that will not come.

Our holiday came to an end, and we returned to Mathura to leave our children with Perrin. This was the first time we had ever traveled without them, but my misgivings disappeared when I saw them utterly at ease in the luxury of the general's house, surrounded by my sister's love and concern.

We took the train to Bombay and flew to New York via Paris. This was our first time in Paris, which was to become Amir's favorite city in the world. We returned to its symmetry, chestnut trees and long, long walks, weaving in and out of the *ponts* along the Seine many, many times. In December 2001 we spent our wedding anniversary in Paris, eating and living extravagantly. Dinner at Alain Ducasse, a ridiculous but memorable event. Amir would undergo a sea change at this type of restaurant. From opinionated and worldly he would be reduced to putty in their hands, agreeing meekly to eat and pay a ransom for things he didn't even like. The only thing that would bring back his usual spirit would be if there was even a shadow of a suggestion that anything was beyond our financial reach. Then he would order two of that to prove he was the son of a poor man. I found the dinner ridiculous while it was happening, but wonderful in retrospect. And one evening, a rapturous concert by the electrifying pianist Andre Watts and another by Ravi Shankar on the sitar—*sat tar*, seven strings. We had to travel to Paris to hear this native of India. Over my protests, Amir bought me the softest-of-soft black Parisian winter coats, which I now cry into.

Our first experience of Kennedy Airport was beyond bewildering, a town in itself, and we were convinced of the wisdom of making this 'familiarizing' trip before we did it for good with our children. A wickedly expensive cab ride took us across one of the fabulous bridges of New York into Manhattan, to the now-disappeared New Yorker Hotel on 8th Avenue and 34th Street. In our tiny room on the thirtieth floor, we caught our first glimpse of the Hudson River, on whose banks thirty years later we would make our last home together.

The grid pattern of Manhattan allowed us easy understanding and access. Amir did not take well to standup eateries, and he exploded when he discovered what was meant by the SRO sign in theatres. We saw several musicals, which I later discovered were a total waste of time for me—I did not remember them minutes after we had walked out of the theatre. But we did see that exuberant, irrepressible, funny and poignant 'Hair.' We saw it again with the children. 'The Age of Aquarius' still sits in an affectionate part of my heart.

The trip to Brooklyn was sobering. The frugally furnished two-bedroom apartment which was to be our home for the next two years, after our African splendor, was daunting. But we had bottomless energy and were refreshed by wandering into nearby Prospect Park and the Botanical Gardens. These gorgeous spaces would be my children's backyard, and the magnificent Brooklyn Museum and Public Library their learning ground. They would lose their free and open African game parks, but this, I romanticized, was their passport to civilization. Yes, this was fine and we were ready.

And it was springtime. Two dainty miniature magnolia trees bloomed at the sides of the stone lions guarding the New York Public Library. Masses of tulips adorned the median of Park Avenue. Fields of daffodils were naturalized into Central Park. An outsized Alice sitting on a toadstool in the company of the Mad Hatter, the poor dormouse who was dunked into the teapot, the forever late white rabbit, the Cheshire cat and the caterpillar. And children clambering all over this bronze statuary at the side of the boating pool in Central Park. I couldn't wait to bring my children to Alice, who was their and my good friend.

We shopped at Gimbel's and bought some basic cook and dinnerware. That night we were to dine at the home of a doctor who had been our classmate. He had emigrated to the U.S. soon after his residency and subspecialized in pediatric genetics. We were surprised to see the insulated traditional Moslem household he maintained, but his family was warm and welcoming and we left our purchases with them.

We also visited another medical-school classmate, one of Amir's original Mafia brotherhood—Indru Khubchandani—in Allentown, Pennsylvania. He had emigrated there in the early years and qualified as a colono-rectal surgeon. His palatial house—they have since moved to an even more overwhelming manor—was seemingly equipped with every luxury. He summed it up by saying his American dream was a king-sized bed, an electronic garage opener (for his three-car garage) and an ice-making machine. These seem humble compared to the material splendor he presently enjoys.

We spent some more time in Brooklyn, meeting our future chiefs, mine the tall aquiline-featured gentle Englishman Dr. Clemetson and Amir's the acerbic Dr. Charlie Pryles, who maintained his home on Pinkney Street in Boston where he returned for weekends by the Boston/N.Y. shuttle plane. This was our first glimpse of lives where distances meant little.

Dr. Clemetson was a total misfit in the essentially clinical service he ran, leading a group of typical private obstetrician/gynecologists who held him in considerable scorn. The money ethic had not pervaded him, and his consultants looked down on him for that. He was an expert on ascorbic acid and, like his guru Linus Pauling, was regarded as a nut in this area as he tried to spread the feeling that much in life depended on this vitamin. He took me to his mouse lab and promised me I cannot remember what if I spent time there. I recklessly agreed, even though the thought of proximity to these vermin gave me the creeps.

A year later when I was working with him, he took me to a dinner meeting of the New York Obstetric Society at the Yale Club in Manhattan. As we walked back to his car, he gave me tips on successful living in New York. Amongst them were always to beware of people in sneakers (about 90 percent of the population) as they could noiselessly creep up on you. Then he really disgusted me by asking me to guess what was concealed in his the breast pocket of his jacket. When I said I didn't have a clue, he unbelievably drew out a can of mace, saying this was essential equipment. I removed him from my worthy list where he had been featured till then.

Rendezvous in Cairo

It was time to return for our rendezvous in Cairo with Perrin and the children. We flew as scheduled to Paris, but the United Arab Airways flight from Paris to Cairo was nowhere to be seen. It finally arrived and with trepidation we arrived in Cairo four hours later than our planned meeting. It was the early hours of the morning, and there was no sign of Perrin and our children. We checked at the airport hotel with no luck. The dead-of-night airport was only alive with shifty characters trying to sell us currency and cigarettes. One such man came up to us and before Amir could spurn him, he asked me if we were looking for a woman who looked like me with three children in tow. I almost fainted, but clutched onto him as he hailed a friend taxi-driver who drove us to the innards of Cairo.

Just as we started to get very uneasy, he stopped at a hotel and accompanied us to the third floor. We knocked, and there the darlings were. Perrin was beside herself with anxiety as apart from everything else, the Indian government at the time only allowed the equivalent of ten dollars to be taken out of the country. She had wisely rationed it out with pure treats, eschewing all real food, so as to divert attention from her anxious situation. So we found our lost children in this congested Cairo hotel, peaceful and content with candy and coca-cola. We gathered them up and all five of us slept in one bed, allowing Perrin to luxuriate deservedly in lone splendor in the other one.

The next day we hurried to the UAA desk at the airport and were not surprised that the next plane to Kampala was not until the following day. We went back to the hotel and slept till evening, and then decided to go to the *son-et-lumiere* held every night at the Giza pyramids.

Amir and I had been warned about the evil ways of the local taxi-drivers, so we acquired a street map of Cairo and I, since Amir was totally incapable of finding the shortest path between two points, charted the route. We hailed a taxi, and Amir gave him a long talk on the route we wanted to take. The driver yessed us and soon proceeded to take us the way he wanted in spite of Amir's protests. We had lived in the city for some hours and he, the taxi driver, dated back to the Pharaohs, but we knew better. When we arrived at the pyramids Amir was livid and did not tip the man.

We attended the outstanding show—beautifully and mournfully intonated with deep glimpses of past lives on a heroic scale—that silvery silent desert with a half-moon glinting on the ruined nose of the Sphinx.

At the end of the show all three children were fast asleep. Amir carried Rushna, I Cena, and Perrin carried baby Sharyn. On coming out there was only one taxi, and it was the same man who had brought us. I had a deep foreboding, but Amir gave him a long lecture and told him he would only get paid if we were taken by the shortest route.

The taxi driver had a look on his face that solidified my uneasiness. He told Amir to rest the children and women in his car and then led him around to the open trunk. In it lay my handbag.

I had left my handbag in the taxi with every document, passports, airline tickets, checkbook, travelers' checks and cash. I never missed it once at the show. If it were not for the driver's fine character, we might still have been wandering the streets of Cairo, paperless penniless paupers.

At our hotel, the newly chastened Amir invited the man in for a drink. 'I am a *chust* Moslem,' he said, and alcohol had never touched his lips, 'but I and my family do eat.' Thoroughly humbled, Amir gave him a handsome tip.

We found our children in an impossible city and were saved from pauperdom, all by the good will of poor men.

Last days

The things one accumulates over time—mostly of no consequence. The business of daily life is untidy. Sharyn was still fond of her dolls, and it became of major concern which to take and which to continue life in Africa. She entrusted the ones who were to stay in the able hands of Elena, who promised to care for them through teen age, middle age and old age. Our house had a small book-lined study. Which to leave behind? We picked enough to fill two cartons of books from the childhood of my girls and those from the years when Amir and I read almost indiscriminately. Private practice years had the advantage of free time to indulge this passion. I now read from those same books to my grandchildren and regale them with poems from the exquisitely illustrated *Oxford Book of Children's Poetry*. I can remember a touching one that I would recite with my children and now recite with my grandchildren.

'Four ducks in a pond,
A blue sky beyond,
White clouds on the wing,
Such a little thing
To remember for years
To remember with tears!'

If I saw agitation at leaving, four ducks in a pond would quiet the nervous hearts.

I recently looked for books that dated from the Africa years.

An Area of Darkness by now-Nobelist V.S. Naipaul introduced to us and inscribed by Daphne Kayton, who delivered my firstborn. This acerb confused us, as I said, by accepting knighthood. Sir Vidya! An old hardback copy of *Pnin*, one of the more obscure novels of Nabokov. It still has a Uganda crested crane logo and asserts that it is the property of the Uganda Public Library. Hopefully, I bought it and did not just walk off with it. J.D. Salinger's 'Raise High the Roofbeam...' Whenever a Tejani was to do something daunting, at least one message of encouragement would read, 'Raise high the roofbeams, carpenter, a Tejani is on her way'. The book is dated 21/9/68 in Amir's small careful script. What could have happened on that day? 'What did one wall say to the other?' Answer: 'Meetcha at the corner.' Or was that in 'Esme'? How we loved that dysfunctional Glass family. I reread *Catcher in the Rye* later when Rushna was a restless teenager and hated Holden Caulfield's pure and simple delinquency. What I had previously thought enchanting made me shudder when my teenager was trying hard to be everything she was not.

And then there were African staples, *Born Free*, Alan Paton's *Cry the Beloved Country*. And Alan Moorehead's *No Room in the Ark*, replete with luscious black-and-white photographs of East African wildlife with clichetic titles that did them no justice. I see that I bought that book for 25 cents.

I note with some guilt that I had never acquired a library of African writings—of which there were many.

We did take some oil paintings of Kampala artists, which still adorn my walls. Also a fragile almost transparent blue-and-white Chinese dinner set, made even finer by embedded rice-grain impressions, which arrived in the U.S. reduced to fine talcum powder. Why would any family with the stress of leaving a life behind and starting in strange lands anew need a fine Chinese dinner set?

One carton that we never saw in the U.S. contained a sumptuous tortoise that Rushna had created on fabric in an after-school art class she attended. The class was run by a Mrs. Adams in the lush garden of her home on Mbuya Hill. Mrs. Adams had dark short hair and the glowing open face of one who knew more than others. She and her family had adopted the Baha'i faith and attended the

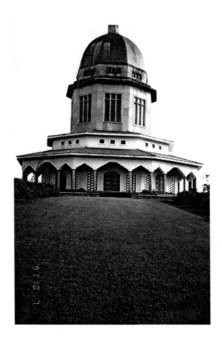

green and gold temple on one of the Kampala hills. Once while waiting for Rushna to gather her things I asked why there was such a relatively large number of Baha'is in Kampala. She told me that a careful reading of the writings of the prophet Baha'i-ulla indicated that he felt that the world was heading toward certain destruction and the only safe haven that would be left was Africa! Poor Africa. Of all the descriptions to apply to it, safe haven verges on cruel and cynical.

Perrin was an inveterate packer. With her husband in the army, she had moved innumerable times. And she said this was always a blessing because it helped shed old baggage and allowed one to start light again. And it was only because of her vetting what we 'could not part with' that we shipped only ten cartons of our belongings rather than many more. If I were to do it again, I would take only photographs and books.

The job done, Perrin left for her home in Mathura, and we moved from our house to Ma's for the final week. We said our goodbyes in large and small gatherings. Bella and Len had left before us. We bid the Kingdons goodbye at Laila and Aneel's place. On our last night we put the children to sleep with Ma and went with our friends Anil (a chest physician in Cairns, Australia) and Nalini (who wrote the Hansards, the minutes of the parliamentary proceedings, for Obote's government) Patel. We had dinner at the only French restaurant in town, Chez Joseph. Said goodbye to Joseph. On to the Susanna night club, and dancing to a lively and natural beat. And then we took a late late-night grand walking tour of the central part of the city. Past the parliament buildings, the National Theatre, the Apollo Hotel and the gardens heavy with green containing the Independence monument, a woman breaking her swathing bondage and holding aloft a baby. Peaceful living would be so easy if it came from art.

We arrived back at Ma's place, but our friends, specially Anil Patel, were reluctant to say goodbye. They sat in the small living room continuing to drink whatever, Scotch, I think. I was quite apprehensive about the reaction of Ma, a chronic insomniac, to the drunken noise from her living room. In spite of my requests, Anil continued to announce loudly how much he was going to miss us. As I tried to smother him, he said he needed to use the bathroom. Well, I thought that would at least keep him quiet for a while, but

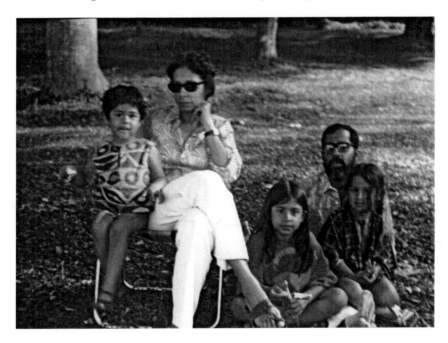

within a minute there was an earth-shaking crash causing everyone in the house to run to the bathroom to see what had happened. Anil emerged from the bathroom and instead of some sort of explanation as to the crash, to Ma's indignation, he just reiterated with his arms around us and endearing tears in his eyes, how he would miss us. We finally helped him into his car, and Nalini drove him home.

It is difficult to remind myself, as I write, that when we said goodbye to family and friends in June of 1971, most had no thought of ever leaving Uganda. November of 1972 found them all devastated and scattered to the corners of the earth, many reunited with us.

EIGHT

Arrival in the USA

To the airport

On the way to the airport at Entebbe on July 3, 1971, we stopped at Bapa's brother Badru's place to say goodbye to his family, but especially to Amir's aging grandmother, whom we would never see again. I wept when she quietly did to my children what she had done to me years ago in Fort Portal when she had first met me. She put her cool hand on their heads and gave each of them a few Uganda shillings. When we got the news of her death a few months later, I was with the children on Sixth Street in Brooklyn, just coming back from the grocery store. Amir came toward us and gave us the news. Sharyn, aged three, startled us by throwing herself on the sidewalk, sobbing inconsolably. She said she remembered the moment that the venerable lady had blessed her with her hand and given her the precious shillings. And she admonished us, saying such news should never be given to someone who was only three years old.

We drove to the airport in a caravan of cars. As we assembled in the lounge I saw all the faces that had come to meet me at the railroad station eleven years before when I had first set foot in Uganda. The same sea of faces. Only now they all had a story, a heart, a soul, to give meaning to the faces.

Amir's mother had to say goodbye to him yet another time. Her first goodbye was when he went as a pre-teenager to the Aga Khan Boarding School in Dar-e-Salam. Amir often remembered that he did not know how to tie his shoelaces when he went. This was because he had acquired his first pair of laced shoes just before he left, and his mother was too heartbroken to teach him and just tied them for him. Next she bid him goodbye to go to college in Bombay, followed by medical school in Bombay. And now, when she thought she had him for life, he was off again. No matter, mother—Idi Amin will make sure that you see him again, soon.

Ma did not tolerate this goodbye well, and her usually smiling face was a tragic mask. We said goodbye in circles, the circle always beginning and ending with her.

We walked down the tarmac when our flight was announced, and I turned once to see the sad but smiling faces. I noted with astonishment that my children skipped ahead with nary a backward glance. A lesson. Amir was smiling and had on his excited look. There was not a shred of apprehension in the five of us. Youth imparts a kind of foolish confidence.

My children were seasoned travelers, and they had a settling-down routine in planes. Three-year-old Sharyn would 'read,' eat and then snuggle with her personal blanket and a pacifier that she still used. As she nuzzled the blanket I saw she had no pacifier. To my surprised look, she told me that her sister Rushna had told her that pacifiers were illegal in the U.S., and the two of them had taken a pair of scissors to her stock. I glared at Rushna, who glared back at me. No trauma, hurt or harm came from this.

We arrived at Heathrow Airport and planned to spend the evening with Pheroze, Amir's brother, who was in London. He met us when we landed, and we had dinner together. Pheroze was always a big favorite of the children. Amir and I had worked every Saturday morning and he, a student at Makerere College, would take them out. They had a routine—Savji brother's toy store and then Christo's bakery for a treat. The smell of that Greek bakery on a Saturday morning has stayed with me. No other bread was warmer or homier. After Pheroze had finished his bachelor's degree, his sociology teacher had financed him on a trip to Karamoja in the arid north of the country, to study the ways and customs of the ancient Karamojong people. Pheroze did not have this burning need to know more about the Karamajong and soon abandoned the project, its incomprehensible people, language and land. Both feet on familiar ground is where he was most comfortable.

Years later Amir had a similar routine with our granddaughter

Tehmina, who would come to us on Sundays and stay through Monday. I would be working, but Amir's job had enough flexibility to take her to the local arcade in Ossining. First the toy store, where a random plastic extravaganza was acquired, the bigger the better. Then the pet store replete with snakes, mice, fish, guinea pigs, exotic silken eared rabbits and blue-hued wicked-looking macaws who said 'Hello, hello.' And then on to McDonald's for chicken nuggets and french fries.

When we left Pheroze at Heathrow Airport we felt we had cast away the last bridge to the old world.

First days in America

We arrived at Kennedy the afternoon of July 5th, 1971, and entered our apartment in Brooklyn just opposite the Methodist Hospital where I was to work for the next two years in the evening. Loud fireworks greeted us, and I had to disillusion the children that they were not to mark our arrival, but were the aftermath of American Independence Day the day before.

We left our children with Dr. Kofi Amankwah, a Ghanian physician who was to be my chief resident, and went to fetch our pots and pans from Dr. Qazi. We were soon back, and Rushna and Amir walked over to the grocery store across the street. It seems incredible, but having left a country, our lives, behind, we didn't miss a beat, ate bacon and eggs for dinner and were soon in bed.

The next morning the children went to summer camp at a local Montessori school, and Amir and I walked several miles to Atlantic Avenue to acquire a car. I have made some good decisions in my life, but this was not one of them. I insisted we buy a no-frills stick-shift inexpensive car—the infamous Cricket.

There was always a vacant parking spot on Sixth Street just in front of the apartment building. Amir convinced himself and me that things were so organized in the U.S. that the spot had been created for us. Our parking problems seem to have been solved till one of the residents asked me if my husband and I had a special dispensation to park in front of a fire hydrant!

We next went to the utterly dreary and crowded Department of Motor Vehicles to obtain U.S. driver's licenses. After waiting hours,

Amir saw a board which posted the countries where reciprocity was accepted without having to go through the road test again. Uganda was not on the long alphabetical list, and just as we were about to turn away, I saw handwritten at the bottom of the list 'UGANDA.' Thus we painlessly got our U.S. licenses and thus I never, to this day, have learned to parallel park.

Soon after we acquired the Cricket, we were invited to a barbecue at the home of one of Amir's attendings in Long Island. While driving back in the dusk, we realized that the car's headlights were not working. Just as we turned the corner for our apartment, a child rushed out into the street and was hit by our car. She was petrified but unhurt, and we did what we would have done in Africa, just carried her into the hospital Emergency Room. The child was upset but physically well, her parents materialized from somewhere and actually thanked us for bringing their daughter to the emergency room. A few days later two tough-looking detectives came to the apartment saying we had left the scene of the accident. We pleaded ignorance successfully.

The Cricket's problems did not end there. When it rained, the car flooded. When we complained, the rascally dealer said all American cars leaked! Finally on a trip to Allentown, Pennsylvania, it died, and we traded it in for an oversized green Ford station wagon and have had one of those gas-guzzlers ever since.

The trip to Allentown was memorable as it was our first experience with tolls. As we stopped at the toll booth, a ticket spewed out at us. I guessed we should just take it and see what happened. But Amir with his suspicious mind said, 'How does it know where we are going?'

To the chagrin of the occupants in the line of cars that was forming behind us he yelled 'Allentown, Allentown' into the unmanned ticket dispenser. We finally got the message.

Relearning the trade

I was a third-year resident in a twelve-person residency. The other eleven were a United Nations of physicians from India, Pakistan, Indonesia, Iran and Nigeria—international graduates as they are now euphemistically called. The door is presently shut to these folk with the loss of some really bright people who were the academic and research backbone of U.S. obstetrics. The only U.S. nationals in the program were two males who had graduated from a foreign medical school in Italy. My first rotation was three months in the Emergency Room with rotational night-call in the labor and delivery unit. It was a decent way to ease myself into practice in this country.

Of course it meant nothing to anyone that I had already earned the MRCOG, the only specialist degree in Obstetrics and Gynecology available in East Africa and that it satisfied all British requirements. Here I had to work toward the American equivalent, the FACOG, Fellow of the American Board of Obstetrics and Gynecology.

At first I had no time to rue being junior to individuals far less experienced or knowing than myself. I had to learn the jargon. My teachers were *attendings*, not *consultants*. I had to learn *elevator* instead of *lift*, *demerol* instead of *pethidine*. No more *foetus*. Even *scrub* nurse instead of *scrubbed* nurse set me apart. I had to stop performing caesarean sections and do cesareans instead. And it took a long time to put the month before the day when writing the date.

And the way the locals spoke! On one occasion, I was obtaining an obstetric history from a young woman who, in response to my question of how many pregnancies she had, said 'I never had no babies.' Two negatives made a positive so, to her great annoyance, I repeated the question. I quickly learnt that two negatives were additive and did not cancel each other out.

In my first week in the Emergency Room a fresh-faced rosy-cheeked schoolgirl came in with her mother and grandmother who said the girl had excruciating abdominal pain. The ER physician called me into the room just in time to deliver this bonny eight-pound baby. The girl was (genuinely, I think) amazed at the sudden abating of her pain and looked at me and asked, 'What was that?' 'A baby boy,' said I. Her smile reassured me that she was not completely in the dark. The mother and grandmother entered the room thinking I had miraculously cured her since the moaning had stopped. On seeing what was in her arms the grandmother passed out and had to be resuscitated in the adjoining ER booth.

Summer school

At summer school, the children had an undemanding routine of reading, writing, peanut butter and jelly sandwiches, cookies, swimming and resting. And the artwork. It is amazing how children the world over draw the same sunny pictures. I was once looking at a book compiled of children's art from the concentration camps of Terezin. None of the children survived, but there were the pictures. The same sun, blue skies, trees, flowers and Mama. The very same pictures my children drew in Africa and now on this Western shore.

The children would arrive home at three in the afternoon, and I had arranged with the wife of an internal medicine resident to meet them and let them into the apartment. At 3.30 p.m. in would come a young babysitter, a great bear of a boy, the son of Mrs. Callaghan, the head nurse in the ER, who played and romped with the children. I often found him exhausted when I got back at 6. Amir and I arranged that we were never on call the same night. So he and I saw each other sporadically and often only in passing. What sustained us? A fierce need to make it all work.

I had a fall-back emergency system for the children. I had given Rushna the telephone number and the name of an ER nurse who agreed to page me in an emergency. One afternoon I knew the babysitter was going to be late, and I got a call from the ER nurse who told me to go home as there was an emergency as reported by Rushna. I was at a conference on the 7th floor of the hospital. I ran down the seven floors, across the street and up the three floors to the apartment.

Rushna and Cena greeted me at the door and said some inconsequential teasing had occurred. Sharyn, whose passions were well known, went into one of the bedrooms and slammed the door, and now the door couldn't be opened by any of the sisters. I looked down at the slobbery mess on the floor. Rushna hastened to explain that they did not let her starve to death or die of thirst. Sharyn had announced that she was hungry, so the others had squashed up grapes and shoved them under the door, and when she said she was thirsty they flung water under, too. The recipient of all this largesse, on the other side of the bedroom door, was lapping up the food and drink from the floor. This despite the fact that she'd had a hearty meal two hours before.

I told Sharyn to stand clear of the door and with a mighty kick flung it open. The reunited sisters hugged and kissed each other as after a long and painful absence.

School started in September, and on the advice of others, the girls were enrolled into private schools. Brooklyn public schools were a drug market, we were told. Rushna and Cena went to the Berkeley Institute, and Sharyn continued pre-kindergarten at the Montessori School. The first week of school I took a vacation so I could be there for their departure and arrival in yellow school buses.

But the rest of the day was mine and I visited New York as a tourist. The great Metropolitan Museum niched into Central Park, the Museum of Modern Art with its water-lily room. The Guggenheim like the inside of a snail shell and the Cloisters, an eclectically situated medieval museum in a 'lifted' monastery with garden courtyards full of Shakespearean herbs and ancient plants—all overlooking the big gray George Washington Bridge and the little red lighthouse of story.

And I observed the vast riches of Fifth and Madison Avenues, and the homeless people who also belonged.

A deeper difference in culture

After I had adjusted to the routine on the Obstetrics and Gynecology service, I realized there were deeper differences that were harder to learn.

I gulped as I watched and then administered the amnesic agent scopolamine and the occasional 'bad' reaction, with the patient growing utterly wild, requiring restraints. The next day, amazingly, the patient complained of bruising where she had been restrained, but had no recollection of the whole episode. What trusting women these are, I thought to myself, trusting in their paternalistic obstetricians—almost exclusively older white males at the time. They had no memory of the birth process, but accepted the stranger baby given to them the next day. The degree of sedation used in labor made me unable to relax, and I was constantly checking for signs of life—they looked so out of it.

I came from a cesarean section rate of 3% in Uganda to the U.S. rate in the 1970's, which was 16-18%. All complicated vaginal delivery had been abandoned, though some of the older obstetricians used Barton's forceps, with a hinged blade, with great skill. One of my wedding presents had been a pair of Kielland's forceps, a beautiful sleek instrument with a sliding lock to accommodate asynclitism — tilting — of the fetal head, and no pelvic curve to allow rotation of the blades with minimal maternal injury. I had brought these forceps to the U.S. — just in case. Since they saw no use, I relegated them to the kitchen, where they were extraordinarily useful in reaching and bringing down unreachable objects. At one teenage party in our subsequent home in Long Island, they disappeared. I can only guess at the use they have been put to by one of Rushna's friends.

At a conference one afternoon to discuss a patient who had a critical medical problem and who was to have a repeat cesarean section, since vaginal birth after cesarean section was taboo, I timidly suggested allowing the woman to deliver vaginally, thus saving her anesthesia and a surgical procedure. This was the first of the 'In this country...' responses I suffered, with the clear implication that in the bush where I came from, things were different and I had better learn the ways of the country I was now in.

And it was true that I had much to learn of local mores, but as the year progressed I had a different problem. I learned to hold to a fine line where I felt I had more experience and knowledge than senior residents and some of the younger attendings. I learned to hesitate before action, to wait to be told what to do before doing it. A strange spot to be in — in a place unsuited to my level of practice. Years later I read a poem by American poet William Matthews who in another context explained my feelings and those of many in my position:

'Don't play too much,
don't play too loud,
don't play the melody.'

Just slide around and draw no attention. I had to deal with three chief residents. One was Dr. Kofi Amankwa, the Ghanian physician who had sheltered the children on our first day in the country. He was a small but heavy-set person with twinkling eyes and constant ideas of new ways to look at things. When I was on call at night with him he never slept and expected that I would not as well while he would talk to me of dozens of alternative ways to look at a problem. He subsequently, like me, did a sub-specialization in Maternal–Fetal medicine and now practices in a teaching situation in Canada. We meet occasionally at the national meetings, and grayer and older as we both are, he is still talking and full of ideas.

The second chief resident was an Indian woman who seemed to take an immediate dislike to me and showed this in word and deed. As inexplicable as this was, her attitude literally changed overnight and suddenly she became a fawning sycophant who acknowledged my superior experience whenever she could. I could not figure either attitude, but certainly preferred the latter.

The third was a Korean, Dr. Kim. Pleasant, surgically talented and quiet, he seemed to be able to handle me just right, like the baby bear interacting 'just right' with Goldilocks. Later, I realized the reason. He, too, was from a background of experience and skill and had to tone things down to fit the role of trainee. He recognized this in me, and we were a harmonious duo. He and I enjoyed performing cesarean sections together, and he would boast to others that if he assisted, with Tejani as the surgeon, no cesarean section could last more than twenty minutes—'skin to skin.'

Saved by Thorazine

Another obstetric cultural shock I sustained when I first arrived in New York in 1971 was the question all laboring mothers were asked—barked at—at a time when labor was engulfing them. 'Breast or bottle?' demanded the nurse. And almost all weakly responded 'Bottle.' Delivery was followed by medications containing high doses of estrogen to suppress lactation. When these drugs were discovered to have high risk for clotting in the veins, they were abruptly withdrawn and the usual nihilism was used instead. 'My breasts are killing me, doctor.' That's life, honey. An affirmation of 'Bring forth your young in sorrow and pain.' Some such biblical adage.

With time fashions have changed and the breast is 'in,' with the usual North American trappings. A lactation specialist on every maternity floor. Lactation consultants available on the telephone for a fee. Charge nurses on the postpartum floors were required to report results of this flurry of activity. Once, in an idle moment, I asked to see these numbers and was told that the breast feeding rate had jumped to 90%. On questioning how long the patients were followed, I was told 'till discharge'! Which was 24-48 hours for a vaginal delivery and three days for a cesarean section. How much paper, how many trees have been sacrificed to these ridiculous 'studies' and reports.

In Uganda of the '60s it was recognized that there was no option. It was breast feeding or death for the baby of the indigent woman. In the absence of clean water, unprocessed cow's milk diluted with river, well or 'puddle' water was a deadly combination. To the rescue came pharmaceutical companies providing infant formulae at subsidized rates. The death formula persisted because although the formulary powder was clean, water used to reconstitute the milk remained the same. Mothers bringing in dehydrated little bundles of bones held together by a lax waxen skin, gastroenteritis and dehydration beyond help were a daily occurrence.

Recent reports show that formula-fed babies in Uganda have the same hazards as four decades ago. It is customary in HIV/AIDS-infected mothers to proscribe breast feeding as there is a chance of passing the infection to baby in breast milk. However, in Uganda this serious consequence is less likely to occur than death from gastroenteritis in formula-fed babies. The recommendation is therefore to breast feed and risk the chance of HIV transmission.

Ugandan mothers were exhorted to breastfeed for a year. The familiar sight of a baby in a bright cloth sling over the mother's chest—often fastened tightly to the breast, or in a hammock on her back with dark hair and bright eyes peeping out—were a necessity to the breastfeeding dictum. A waning milk supply in a woman who had to take to the fields, tend the *shamba*, cook on an open fire, and sell her wares at the weekly market in the city several miles away was common.

A professor from Tulane enunciated the thorazine cure. I can vouch for the enormous milk-enhancing properties of this medication. When about 28 weeks into my first pregnancy, I took a tiny dose for gastritis. I was surprised twelve hours later to find myself flowing with milk—still safely pregnant. The Tulane professor had an unforgettable wife who was a familiar figure in Kampala. She had a helmet of blond hair and fingernails painted bright black, the same as my granddaughters do now. A woman before her time.

Thorazine became part of the send-off package for delivered women. A pathetic little package containing a few muslin diapers, safety pins to hold them together, a small can of Baby Johnson's talcum powder, clean dressings for the umbilical cord stump…and thorazine. When a woman came for her six weeks postpartum visit, one of the questions would be on the continued use of thorazine. Very matter of fact—have you taken your thorazine?

A note about the Baby Johnson talcum powder. In my time this was an essential for child rearing. Its nostalgic odor has forever become part of the 'baby' smell for me. We have cast this away because of suspicions of inhaling it and causing lung disease and being associated with future ovarian cancer in girl babies. Just cannot believe or stomach these reports.

Back to the thorazine story. Thorazine is a psychotropic drug with multiple uses and an array of side effects. A standard reference says the following for its use in nursing mothers: 'There is evidence that chlorpromazine (thorazine) is excreted in the breast milk of nursing mothers. Because of the potential of serious adverse reactions in nursing infants from chlorpromazine, a decision should be made whether to discontinue nursing or discontinue the drug…'.

This was before the great 'evidence-based' days. What could have happened? Generations of addicted babies? 'Good' babies who slept and slept and never cried. Slow babies? But definitely babies who survived because of their mothers' overflowing milk. A THORAZINE generation.

Thanksgiving and Christmas

Amir brought home with him a co-resident, Venketesan Krishnan, who lived with his sister Vijaya Venketesa in an apartment in Brooklyn Heights. Last name usage amongst South Indians is incomprehensible, as illustrated by this pair. However, Krishnan had an encyclopedic knowledge of just about everything from trivial upwards—'the largest clover-leaf in the world is just before entering Death Valley,' the vagaries of the 'windchillfactor,' which he pronounced as one word, the beauty of Harlem streets. Krishnan became a friend who helped us bridge many many valleys, streams and mountains on our way to understanding and being understood.

His sister Vijaya was a black-eyed beauty who said she was a psycho-linguist. Later, she decided this was too esoteric and, like us, no one had a clue as to what this meant. She applied to law schools and was accepted into NYU. On the first day of school, she realized that she had been accepted into a postgraduate program and there was no open place in the basic first year of law school. She gave it some thought and decided to accept the position! After six months, when she was excelling, she confessed to one of her teachers, who let her continue, saying she could use the postgrad qualification after she had properly qualified. So she became the first lawyer in history who obtained her postgraduate qualification in international law and became a regular lawyer later. She eventually graduated from law school in London and has lived there ever since.

When our first November in this country rolled around, everyone prepared for Thanksgiving. Amir and I would have this holiday off and work over Christmas, the usual trade-off. Since we had no sense or feeling for the occasion, we agreed to Krishnan's suggestion to drive north, find an inn to eat at and take our first view of New York State. So the five of us with Krishnan and Vijaya piled into our station wagon and drove up through the borough of Queens, over the Whitestone Bridge crossing Long Island Sound. Further east, we saw its identical twin, the Throgs Neck Bridge. Then into the Bronx and Westchester County. We crossed the Hudson at its widest point over the Tappan Zee Bridge, which Krishnan told us connected the older villages of Tappan to the east and Zee (incorrectly) to the west. And then further and further north to Bear Mountain.

We stopped at a little inn, warm and comfy with wood-burning stove and the smell of apples and cinnamon. After a turkey meal, we walked to a nearby gentle slope and, intoxicated by the cold crisp weather, we practically ran to the top. As we descended the gentlest of snowflakes touched us and the children knew they were snow queens. As we came to the base of the slope we heard a loud rustle and out of the woods came two hunters with their guns at the ready. They astonished us by saying they had thought we were deer and followed us all the way down. I looked at Cena in a fawn-colored coat with large brown deer eyes. The fall hunting season and the American's right to bear arms I had yet to learn and never accepted. But we learned to wear red in October and November when walking the woods.

People call Thanksgiving the dress rehearsal for Christmas. A month later for Christmas, I got a tiny tree, small enough to place on a side table, and the children threaded it with flowers. One of us lit a candle, and all of us howled with laughter as Amir solemnly intoned 'an immigrant's first Christmas.'

1972: Pregnant children

The Obstetrics and Gynecology Service at the Methodist Hospital was largely private with a slew of physicians in private practice caring for their patients with the help of the residents and, in doing so, training them. Some were good practice-based teachers and some were users.

As was the case in most predominantly private hospitals, about twenty percent were publicly supported 'service' patients. One of the few programs run specially for this group was an adolescent pregnancy clinic. Teenage pregnancy was at an all-time high in the country and much time, attention and writing was expended on the problem. Twenty years later the issue is less pressing. But most cynics do not believe it was because of the effort of the 70's and 80's. They feel it was more because the fear of HIV/AIDS caused differences in sexual practices, thus causing teenage pregnancy rates to fall.

Besides teenage pregnancy clinics we all participated in classes for these young mothers. It was my turn one Tuesday afternoon. I always felt discomfited by obviously unwilling students and never have been able to win over dissidents. I function best when my students are adoring sycophants from the start.

My assignment was cesarean section. It was too late to do anything about the real problem, 'children having children.'

Their chances at freedom, school, equipment to make a life were permanently stifled. I looked around for a sympathetic face—one that would nod affirmation when I made a point—one that would encourage me to proceed. My eyes met a few smiley open faces, potential focus points.

'The cesarean section rate in this country is 16%,' I said. 'It is not higher in young people.' It's like athletes—those marvelous teenaged swimmers who roar through water unimpeded by friction or common sense. Labor is an athletic business. The mechanics of it are well handled by our teenaged athletes.

My attention wavered as I saw an unresponsive heavily pregnant visage gazing out the window as a dusting of snow chastened the scene. Where was she? Not with me, for sure.

To continue. 'Failure to progress is the commonest reason for performing a cesarean section.' Unfortunate words, *failure to progress*. Are they thinking that it is a description of their young lives? Obstetric terms are so enslaving. *Labor*, estimated date of *confinement, failure to progress*.

I saw a raised hand at the right of the circle. 'Can my mother be with me?'

'Yes, yes.' Child, are you ever going to connect with the real problem?

'Another common reason for cesarean section is fetal distress.' More unfortunate terms.

'What distresses the baby?'

'Lack of oxygen.'

'Why? How?' I am happy at the sudden interest.

'Impaired placental perfusion.'

Is arrogance preventing me from really explaining? In another setting high school students this age would easily understand that oxygen is transferred across the placenta following the laws of diffusion of gases. But this is a living dynamic situation so other factors play a part. The blood flow through the uterus, the umbilical blood flow, the increased affinity of fetal blood for oxygen, local arrangements of flow. And then there is Fick's principle. That's a simple one. Let me try.

$Ut = F\ (A\text{-}V)$, where
Ut = Utilization
F = Flow
A = Arterial level
V = Venous level

'The utilization of a substance, say oxygen, is expressed by the rate of blood flow times the difference in the concentration of oxygen between the arterial and venous ends.' I have said this sentence countless times—it is one of few biological truths. But today it sounds like incomprehensible nonsense. I regret taking this seemingly elitist route to avoid seeming condescending. I am finding it difficult to just be myself. I have really no connection with the group.

Could it be possible? At the far end of the room there was a pregnant child sucking her thumb and stroking her upper lip with a well-worn blanket. No one else seemed to mind. I forced myself to stop staring.

And a moment ago I was spewing Fick's principle!

'Another reason for cesarean section is malpresentation. For example, if the buttocks of the baby are presenting instead of the head.' The word *buttocks* caused peals of laughter. I was at a loss. Should I scold? Or ignore the laughter and continue with raised voice. I gave up and laughed with them. Look at me now, I thought. I am laughing at the word *buttocks*! But it was a good move. I saw some sympathy.

My eyes wandered back to Ms. Thumbsucker. She was almost asleep. How to appeal to their attention? Shake them with bloody tales of operative technique? Sing them a nursery rhyme? Green eggs and ham?

But this group was shortly to take on motherhood. Soon to be 'emancipated minors.' What does that mean? Drink, drive, be drafted, vote? No, it meant they could sign consent for themselves when they came to the hospital, often unaccompanied.

'Thumbs' was asleep and emitting faint and then louder snoring sounds. This did not amuse or even engage the group. Sleeping was accepted behavior in class.

I began to will my pager to go off for some emergency that I could certainly handle better than this. It did not oblige.

I switched to the Socratic method. 'What is another reason for a cesarean section?'

Answer, 'A baby boy.'

I am perplexed, as is the group. 'Why is that?'

'Because boys is trouble.' A quick look around the classroom affirmed this as a basic truth.

'What else?'

'I'm going to have a cesarean section.'

'Why is that?"

"Because all my children were by cesarean section.'

Health care providers are supposed to show no surprise at human behavior that differs from one's own sense of normality. Non-judgmental always.

But *all* my children in a teenager? I am spared asking the question when someone in the group asked her how many babies she had.

'Two,' she said. 'This is my third. I hope it's a boy. I have two girls.' Even with lightning efficiency, she must have started at age thirteen.

At another such class that I had audited, I remember a kindly and skillful nurse practitioner asking the group their thoughts on pregnancy. After a prolonged silence, I heard some things I will never forget.

'I never thought I could get pregnant.'

'My mother had me when she was twelve.' Shortly to be a grandmother at age twenty-four.

And most piercing, 'I wanted something of my own.'

A visit

A knock at the apartment door in July, and I opened it to see a stranger in patched dirt-gray shorts, a tangled beard reaching low on the chest, modestly covering the gaps and holes in the front of his equally gray tee-shirt. And a mass of knotted hair down his back. He whooped in and hugged me, and the children were delighted to greet and recognize their uncle Mohezin, now a full-blown hippie from hell. I could almost see the lice creeping into Cena's waist-length hair. Before he could spread his gifts around, I dragged him to the bathroom, gave him a brush, antiseptic soap, Kwell shampoo and the children's hair detangler and told him to not emerge for at least an hour. His clothes I threw in the incinerator.

He emerged from the bath smelling like a rose. He, not I, begged me to cut his hair. So I sat him down on the floor and combed and hacked off great masses. He moaned that he felt as demasculated as Sampson and said I was a ruthless Delilah. I was able to comb smooth most of his remaining hair, all except for a massive tangle on the crown of his head. In a fit of frustration, I just lopped it right off. So for a while he went around with this friar's fringe of hair surrounding a near bald patch. It didn't seem to cramp his style at all.

And the children had this jolly companion for the summer days.

A trip across the U.S. and Amin's decree

Amir and I managed to get three weeks vacation in August 1972. I recently read that a person had come to Paris late in his life and felt he could never accept this city that had evolved for so long without him. This is what we felt about the U.S. and thought the quickest review would be to take a three-week cross-country car trip ending in Berkeley, California, where our Uganda friends Bella and Len Feldman lived. From there we would fly home with someone driving the car back for a small price. Mohezin wanted to visit friends in Colorado, so he would accompany us for most of the way.

Our first stop was Washington D.C., where we went to the splendid free museums and monuments. A special moment came when Amir gazed into the eyes of gentle Abe Lincoln and read for the first of many many times his simple and short Second Inaugural Address. On so many future occasions, I have sat at the steps of the monument waiting as he read and re-read those good words.

And, to be well remembered, a permanent protest outside Nixon's fortified White House. We sat on the green park watching, much impressed by this well-tolerated peaceful expression of opposition.

Across the Potomac River, we walked into Arlington National Cemetery to stand by the eternal flame over Kennedy's grave and a white wooden cross marking his brother Bobby's grave. I remembered the day it happened when we had gone into the *charo* and seen simple Ugandan peasants mourning him. '*Mukhade, mukhade'*—'Alas, alas.'

We drove on to the spectacular caverns, caves and secret underground lakes of Roanoke in Virginia. The caverns were on the threshold of the Blue Ridge Mountains and Shenandoah Park. Joan Baez was one of our favorites in Kampala and we knew the Blue Ridge Mountains from her. 'My home's across the Blue Ridge Mountains...and I never expect to see her anymore.' We rolled and walked in the flower-besotted parklands amongst the pines and the flowing water. This country was becoming more beloved by the moment.

We stopped for a night at the at Oconaluftee Village based on the glory that was the Cherokee nation, now reduced to selling trinkets and telling self-conscious stories of the way they thought it had been. That evening we attended an epic open-arena presentation of 'The Trail of Tears,' the story of the mandated move of 15,000 Cherokee from their longtime homes to Oklahoma, legitimized by the villainous treaty of New Echota signed by then-President Andrew Jackson. More than a third of the Cherokee died en route, and where each tear fell to the ground grew a white rose. Too late the tears were honored by proclaiming the White Georgia Rose its state flower.

Although it was a naive production, its innocence brought tears to all of us, specially our passionate Sharyn who wept bitterly and had to be tucked into our sides for protection. Our first year in the country had been all-consuming with no time for reflection. We knew of the native Americans, but the situation did not impinge on us. Suddenly I realized the ruthless life of the primary immigrant, the conquerors, the colonialists reenacted over and over—a battle for survival with the unsuspecting hosts at permanent disadvantage.

We turned west and were soon speeding through the wheat-adorned heartland of the country. We had our pick of sparse townships set in miles and miles of waving and bowing fields, but stopped at Rush (our pet name for Rushna) with a population of fifteen. A hand-painted sign said Coffee Shop, and we asked for ham sandwiches. I saw the proprietress cum waitress cum cook sneak out the back door, go to a grocery store and come back with bread and ham, which she slapped together and served on some really interesting old pottery. We must have been her first customers in eons.

As we left Rush we were tuned to a news station and were jolted into catastrophe. Out there in the American Midwest that had never heard of Uganda, our unbelieving ears heard from the newscaster that Idi Amin of Uganda had a dream the night before. He dreamed that he had been commanded by God to expel all the Uganda Asians as they had 'milked the Ugandan cow without feeding it.' He had also been told by that same God to take over the Asian-owned businesses, properties and possessions. He was to give them 90 days to leave. This was August 5th 1972, the day after the dream. On August 9th 1972 he signed the 90-day ultimatum. November 9th was to be the last date to comply and leave.

Amir's three brothers were out of the country, Mohezin with us, Pheroze in London and Bahadur teaching at the University of Nairobi in Kenya. His parents and his five sisters, all with spouses and children—seven amongst them—were in Uganda. After much discussion, we decided ostrich-like that we could not take this seriously and continued on our trek across the country.

We left Mohezin on a lonely crossroad where he 'knew' he would get a ride on to his friends in Boulder, Colorado. We would miss him, though he did cause us some anxiety when we discovered that his closely guarded backpack contained a pair of purple underpants and a whole mass of cannabis. We made him dump it, and now he was a really light traveler. Just one pair of purple pants and a scowl.

We headed through mountain passes and wild lands to the most scenically glorious state, New Mexico, and stopped at Santa Fe where, if we had spoken Spanish, we would have blended in with the locals. We stopped at the giant Lake Navajo created by the Hoover Dam and then had a brief respite in arty Taos. I could live and love in a place like that.

I had given Rushna an aspirin tablet for a reason I cannot remember and Sharyn, who never wanted to be left out of anything, said she had the exact same problem as Rushna. In an act devoid of commonsense, I gave her one, too. She said she wanted to go to the bathroom soon after, and in a stall in Taos she became ashen and passed out. I cannot remember what I did in panic, but benadryl was involved and she soon came to and has been branded 'allergic to aspirin' for life.'

We continued to Arizona and headed for the Grand Canyon and the Painted Desert. The approach to the parks was filled with neon-rife rows of stores. But all of that disappeared at the park gates, revealing ancient stark canyons set in lonesome beauty. Sharyn was underage to take the donkey trip down to the valley, but we promised it to her at a later time. I remembered the other long-ago trip into the crater at Ngorongoro in another world, another life.

We then left the grandeur of this, our adopted country, and surrendered to Disneyland in Anaheim. The children were wild on rides, haunted houses and various mirages. Somewhere at the back my mind I realized this was unhealthy—but what the hell.

We traveled on to Santa Barbara and had our first look at that vast Pacific Ocean. Black-blue but different from our African waters. Cold, cold and lifeless. We traveled up north through spectacular California Route One, high above the restless ocean on the left and wild places and palatial dwellings on the right.

We reached our friends Bella and Len at Berkeley near San Francisco and after greeting them we asked about Amin and Uganda. They had heard nothing, and we thought we must have dreamt it. Dreamt about Amin's dream.

We arranged for the car to be driven home, and we were to fly back. There was something about Californians. Effusive on the outside and distant and self-absorbed on the inside. I was astounded to realize I missed those gruff but genuine New Yorkers.

We flew back to work and reality. Many messages awaited us from Aneel and Amir's sisters that it was true that they had to shortly leave the country. Most importantly, Ma and Bapa had to have a place. We briefly thought that they would take to India best, but they adamantly refused. So we spent hours at the immigration office doing the necessary for sponsoring them into the United States. When we felt we were up against bureaucracy that we could not handle, Amir wrote to Rep. Edward Koch. Amir addressed him as though he was a United States Senator, and Koch addressed Amir as Professor Tejani (he was a lowly pediatric resident). Whatever Koch's magic was, the papers went through, and on November 12, 1972, Hadibhai Tejani--who was born in India, stowed away on a boat to Africa, and spent a long and worthy life in Kenya, Tanzania and Uganda--arrived in the United States of America. With him was Fatima Tejani, born in Lamu, married at eighteen, who bore nine children and was now entering what was the best, most relaxed phase of her long and passionate life.

NINE

The Sisters' Stories

On the night of August ³ʳᵈ, 1972 in Uganda, which was August 4ᵗʰ in the U.S., as we had learned from American radio, Idi Amin, President of Uganda, had the dream in which he was visited by God, who advised him that the Asian population in Uganda had reached explosive proportions and that he must save the situation. In other accounts, he was also said to have received divine guidance to solve the situation by expelling the Asians and taking over Asian-held assets. He instructed the British ambassador to arrange to repatriate all Indians residing in Uganda with a British

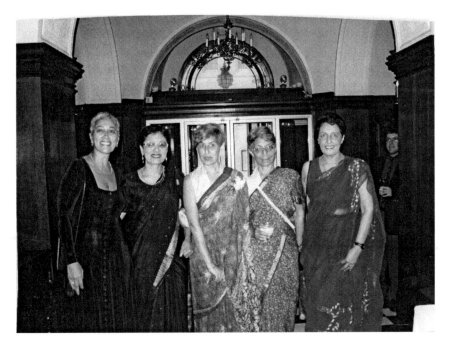

passport. The Indian Government was quick to establish that these individuals were not India's problem and would not accept them. Poor Britain became the most reluctant bride of 50,000 Asians. An official order of expulsion was signed on August 9th 1972 with a deadline of 90 days ending at midnight on November 8th.

As noted, all of Amir's brothers were out of the country at that time. His parents, sisters, their spouses and children were all still there. These are the stories of the sisters, written out in their own words in response to my request and edited lightly by me. This is their account of what happened during those 90 days of turmoil before leaving the continent of their and their mother's birth. Sweet Uganda, goodbye.

Gulshan's story

Gulshan was born in 1935 in Sultanhaud, Kenya, at home, delivered by a lay midwife. She was the second of Ma's surviving children. A premature baby, Khatoon, who died in infancy, was born between Amir, the oldest, and her. In 1957 she married Amir Dhanani, and when I first came to Kampala in January of 1960, she had her first child, a beautiful perfectly round little girl, Shirin or, as she was always called, Shilo. She then had two boys. In 1972 when Amin issued his edict, they were a family of five, recently moved to a beautiful house on Mbuya Hill in Kampala. This is the story of the 90 days between hearing of the edict and their departure from the country where her mother, she, her husband and her children were born.

On Saturday, August 9th, we heard the news of Amin's eviction edict at Laila's brother-in-law Sunil Korde's wedding. We assumed it was another of his whims and could be ignored.

The next morning we heard it was serious and that all persons with Ugandan nationality were to have this verified. If they had not renounced other citizenship within three months of receiving Ugandan citizenship, they would either revert to their original citizenship or be declared stateless. Also, those with British passports would have to confirm the validity of their passports.

The next day, a Sunday, the Ismaili community announced that prayers would be held for a week in the hope that Amin would change his mind. However, not wanting to depend on the power of prayer alone, many people started to move their moveable assets to Kenya and sell off whatever they could not move. Amin soon put a stop to this by sealing the borders and allowing each person to leave with only a thousand Ugandan shillings.

That week I stood in line for hours at the British Embassy to verify our citizenship status. People had been lining up from midnight the night before and there was confusion and a wild rush when the embassy opened for business. Matters were made worse by the unfeeling embassy keeping open for only two hours a day for this purpose, in spite of our obvious desperation. At the end of our wait I was declared a British subject, and my husband Amir was declared stateless. For a reason I cannot remember, three months before, Amir had received a letter saying he was a permanent resident of Uganda. When Amir went to plead his case, he was told to leave the office, threatened by an armed *askari*. He was also told that he was free to leave his three children behind in Uganda since they were born in Uganda!

It was clear that neither the British nor Indian governments wanted this exodus. We had recently moved to a more secluded home on Mbuya Hill. Not having curtains, we kept the lights off at night so as not to attract attention. I went to an Ismaili community leader for advice. He told me to regard myself as a Ugandan and not to leave. And yet a day or two later he had left. There was secrecy among the victims, and very often neighbors would suddenly disappear without a word to us. Our houseboys and ayahs were initially sympathetic, but later appeared to feel they had the upper hand, and I often felt they were spying on us. One day the military police came to Amir's place of work and took him in for questioning on the suspicion that he had sent money out of the country. The summons read Amirali Ebrahim Kassam Dhanani, a name only known to our Asian friends and relatives. We were sure our fellow Asians were informing on us. This was the second brush Amir had with the police. The first was in January, 1971, soon after President Obote had been ousted by Amin. There was a disturbance in our housing complex, and Amir went out to see a woman being dragged into a military jeep. He challenged them and they left him with a large laceration that required thirty-two stitches. We had heard of the disappearance of many prominent Ugandans, so we were happy that he escaped with an injury that quickly healed.

The Aga Khan approached Mr. Trudeau, prime minister of Canada, to help the Ugandan Asians, and a few weeks later Canada set up an immigration center in Kampala. Thousands of Asians applied and were given numbers which were announced in the *Uganda Argus*. Our number, 857, finally was announced. By this time, many were already on their way to Canada. An additional obstacle was that all of us had to obtain a tax clearance verification. When the man in this office asked for a bribe from Bapa, he refused and asked to see his superior, as though order and justice still prevailed. Aneel rescued Bapa by actually paying the bribe. With sponsorship from Amir and Nergesh, Ma and Bapa were processed to them in New York. Our Canadian interview was approved and we were soon to leave for our new home.

We managed to send some of our belongings by ship to friends in Canada. On the day of our departure we were taken to Entebbe Airport by a bus arranged by the Canadians. When the bus took a detour to a newer part of the airport we were certain that this was a trap and we were to be detained and worse. Fear was our constant companion.

There were numerous checks before we boarded. At the first, a family behind us was so jumpy that they tried to jump the line. They drew attention to themselves and were stripped of a large amount of gold they were carrying—probably their life's savings. The officer attending to us kindly told Amir to tell me to go to the bathroom and put my jewelry in my luggage as I might meet the same treatment. I was so nervous that I did it in full view, thus endangering Amir and the officer. When it was my turn to be strip-searched, I heard the woman before me being told that she could only take one ring. I had two and I slipped one under my tongue.

We finally boarded the plane. Amir had tears in his eyes as he left forever the country of his birth and his livelihood. I was obsessed by my children's safety and could only feel relief. In a delayed reaction six months later, I felt my devastating loss.

Amir's sister Sakker's husband would not leave Uganda, so Sakker and her two children left for England without him. She did not hear from him for six months. Finally, as the situation deteriorated, the United Nations ran an airlift taking the remaining Asians to different destinations. Her husband was taken to Malta, and she finally located him there. A year later, he was allowed to join his family.

We felt as though we were embraced by the Canadians. They welcomed us and surrounded us with safety and kindness. Our first stop was Montreal, and then we went to Vancouver. The following day we were at Manpower, the Canadian employment agency. And we ran into my sister Shamim and her husband, Eqbal! We were placed in a home and given a living allowance till we were settled. Amir got a job on the third day—and he never looked back. We are forever indebted to the Canadian government for our new lives and a future for our children.

The scene of Americans leaving Viet Nam haunted me, with mothers begging the last Americans to take their children to the U.S. We left Uganda with our most precious possessions, our children. And although at the time the loss of our material possessions was on our minds, we later realized how lucky we were.

Gulshan and Amir settled in Vancouver. After many partially successful business ventures, they started a business in Bellingham, Washington, just across the U.S.-Canada border, turning old car engines into brand new ones. This venture was so successful that it attracted a giant firm, Yamato, whose need for these engines is seemingly inexhaustible. They now run an establishment employing several hundred people and all three of their children, Shilo, Assiff and Shafique, are part of the business.

Amir's was a real rags to riches story. Incompletely schooled, he started life as a car mechanic. Many failed business ventures followed. And then, stability at last. The couple enjoy their eight grandchildren who live in the vicinity. I just got an invitation to their fiftieth wedding anniversary with a picture of the two when they were just married.

Nisa's story

Born Meher-u-nisa in 1936, in Sultanhamud, Kenya, Nisa was the third of the sibs and the second of the girls, and was called Mary by all except her father, who called her Nisa. Early in her life, she was accident-prone and always crashing into and breaking things—hath bhangli, literally

meaning broken hand, the family called her—till it was discovered that
she was myopic to near blindness. Corrective glasses soon made her enter
the seeing world. Although she was put to work after the fourth grade, she
became an autodidact reader, computer maverick and loans manager.
In 1966 in London she married Salim Faruki, had her first son Mubasher
and returned with her family to Kampala. In 1970, I delivered her of her
second son, Shaqil.
  This is her story of those ninety days.

It was late on a Sunday afternoon that someone—maybe my
neighbor Althea Kironde, an African-American married to a
Ugandan politician—heard over the radio and brought the news
that Amin had declared that all people of Asian origin must leave
Uganda in three months, setting a deadline for November 9th, 1972.
Salim heard the news at a restaurant with friends. When he came
home he had made his decision. 'I am an African (his mother was a
tall, gentle dignified Muganda woman while his father, long dead,
was an Indian), this is my country, we are not going to leave.'

As for me, I was living a life of turmoil, laden with his erratic
outbursts of physical and verbal abuse. I was forever weak,
indecisive and incapable of making changes. Once again, hearing
Salim's decision, I felt afraid and unable to fight what I thought
was a dangerous decision for me and my family. I feared for my
children and remembered the ones I had not allowed to live. At
least they do not feel my pain.

In the days after Amin's decree, regular life for the Asian
community ceased. All who had their papers and the means left.
I buried my head in the thought, 'I am married to an African. I am
staying. This is my country. I am staying.'

I did not miss a day of work. But as September ended there
were visibly fewer Asians in Kampala. Black people on the street
stared at me going about my usual routine while all else was in
turmoil. I gradually realized that staying back was not an option
but had no idea of what to do.

Almost every day Althea brought back news of people she
knew disappearing and of violent deaths. One evening the Indian
boy living across the street ran to us, saying his father had not come
home. Salim went with the boy to look for him without success. The

father's body was found in the neighborhood a few days later. Now it was real. It could be us next.

Amin further tortured our people by qualifying his edict. All Asians did not have to leave. Those with Ugandan citizenship would have their papers 'reviewed.' Many with Ugandan citizenship had presumed being spared, but this announcement drove thousands of Asians with Ugandan citizenship to the Immigration Office, often to wait in lines that lasted all day. If not serviced during working hours, they camped out for the night so as not to forfeit their position in the line. Each day was more chaotic as further obstacles were placed in the path of these people who had decided to become Uganda citizens. One day Salim was in the melee and saw Bapa (my father), already a Uganda citizen, standing in the interminable lines. As he watched, he saw Bapa fainting from heat and stress. Salim helped him to his feet and brought him home.

Soon families and friends were divided. Indian Indians were required to go to India, British Indians to Britain. I fell into the group of 'unqualified' Ugandan Asians because of citizenship granted after 1966 and I was declared stateless. A few, a couple of thousand, Ugandan Asians were declared 'OK' and allowed to stay. Salim, having been born in Uganda, qualified to stay. With that logic, all my sibs and their children should have qualified, but for our color—bright brown. There was no use, time or expectation of success in trying to fight that noble battle.

Salim's official qualification to stay strengthened his decision for all of us to stay.

My father and mother and sisters were all preparing to leave.

Amir and Nergi were already in the U.S. and not here to help. Anxiety gnawed at me into near paralysis, but where children are concerned women have that extra inner strength to push and pull themselves along.

Yet another month passed. That sane and compassionate Canadian government set up a temporary office to interview those declared stateless to ascertain qualification for entry into Canada. My sister Gulshan and her husband Amir had already been accepted into Canada and were in the process of packing crates of what they would take. Their friend Ramzan in Canada was their sponsor. Ma and Bapa were going to Amir and Nergi in New York since they qualified as their dependents. Thank you, someone up there.

I could not stay. Escape, I had to escape. Escape from this now-estranged country of my birth and from my impossible life.

After sleepless nights and daily torment, I went to the Canadian Embassy from work so as to conceal my decision from Salim. On the application form I falsely declared myself to be separated with two children. I wrote that my spouse was part African and did not want to leave, but that I feared for the safety of my children. I qualified on the basis of knowing spoken English, being employable and having a sponsor—also the overloaded Ramzan. How would I work with two small babies they asked. I would find a babysitter, I said, without the slightest idea of life in the west. Suddenly I found myself in tears with people calming me and cooling me with water.

Their wonderfully inviting message was this: 'Come to the embassy any day before the November 9th deadline at 3 p.m.'

'Any day?'

'Yes, any day. Remember only two essentials. Bring your children and bring your passport declaring you stateless. A guarded and armed bus will take you to Entebbe Airport. Air Canada planes are waiting to fly you to safety. Just be there at three.'

I was euphoric till reality suddenly hit me. How was I going to leave without Salim's knowledge? He would take the boys away and force me to stay. He had done that once before. Once after a fight with him, I went to pick Mubasher up from school. His teacher said Mubasher had left with his father. I went home and waited and waited. They did not come home that night. Frantic, I called his brother to take me to Salim's mother's home in Kawempe and found Mubasher there. Salim was at work. Again I caved in and agreed to revert back to 'normal.'

Driving home, I prepared the lie to tell him. I could not ask for help from the Canadian Embassy as I had already made a false declaration to them. I would take Althea into my confidence and ask her to smuggle me and the children out.

I came home but before I could speak Salim told me that his entire family, brothers, cousins, mother were leaving and that I and the children should also leave and he would follow when possible. 'Start working on it,' he told me. With difficulty I kept the appearance of normality. I allowed him to think this was his decision. I said Althea knew people in the Canadian Embassy and she would help me. I ran to Althea's home to tell her of developments.

This was already the first week in November and the deadline was looming. The remaining days are a blur. I ate, slept and even went to work.

I had to be inventive in my cover-up. Every day I came home and recounted what had happened the previous week at the embassy as though it had just happened that day. So everything I said was true, but the timing was off. We decided that our day of departure would be 7th November—twenty-four hours before the deadline.

I packed some clothes for the children, hardly thinking that this was the frigid Canadian autumn. In any case, we had no warm clothes so there was little option.

When the day for departure came, Salim refused to leave us at the embassy to go by the provided bus and said he would drive us to the airport at Entebbe. I was edgy and nervous that something would set him off and he would change his mind about our leaving.

We set off for Entebbe Airport. Mubasher was five and a half years and Shaqil was two. I was determined that once in Canada, I would not let Salim know where I was. I would be out of his life and he out of mine. I was brought back to earth when Mubasher, with his big black eyes and fringed eyelashes, asked Salim, 'When are you coming to join us?' 'Soon, very soon,' he replied and hugged the boys and me. 'Goodbye, goodbye.' I will never see you again.

We were led through an alley of protective red maple-leafed flags, the best use flags have ever been put to. Outside this protective corridor stood the army with guns ready, a terrifying checkpoint. Will my children remember the first time they ever saw a gun, knowing it was aimed at them?

Hundreds of us were herded onto the plane, and suddenly we were surrounded by Canadian stewardesses and stewards consoling our crying children, plying them with soft words, food and miraculous toys. People around me, suddenly released, started talking in Gujerati and English. The talk was astonishingly about what valuables they had salvaged. What about the life and loves we had left behind? Priorities are distorted among the desperate. I was numb and felt nothing. We left Ugandan soil at 7 p.m. on November 7th, 1972.

After a refueling stop at Madrid, we found ourselves in Montreal. We were in light summer clothes in the bitterest of cold with a few inches of snow on the ground—us in sandaled feet. We were driven to army barracks and slept under warm soft blankets. We were OK.

The next morning after a hearty Canadian breakfast we were taken to the army clothing store, where Canadian citizens had donated warm clothing, boots and shoes in all shapes and sizes. Transfixed by snow, Mubasher ran out picked up a snowball and ate it. With frozen hands, he ran back in.

Now that we were properly fed and clothed, the kind Canadians led us to a community hall and started individual interviews to determine how to place us. Their prime objective was to locate family and friends we could start our lives with. My sister Gulshan and possibly Shamim (I was not quite sure of this) were in Vancouver and before the day was out we were on another aircraft headed west to meet them.

It was evening in Vancouver. Volunteer citizens met us and drove us to a motel. The driver settled us in and brought milk for the children. He left saying he would be back in the morning to take us to the Immigration Office to make us legal.

Next morning at the Immigration Office, the unbelievably kind immigration officer welcomed the 200 assembled refugees. He explained that each family would be interviewed to locate local family and friends, find a place to live and start the search for jobs. They would fund us for food, clothing, and day care when I found a job. I would not have to pay for airfare but should arrange to pay back motel rental when a job had been secured. While all this was being explained, the children were being cared for and entertained in an adjoining room. I could not control the tears at such kindness from strangers—nameless people I had never met and whom I would never meet again.

And then, best joy of all, my sister Gulshan's name was located and I called to hear her dear voice. She had an apartment near the Immigration Office and soon came to take us to her home. Mubasher and Shaqil greeted their cousins Shilo, Asiff and Shafiq. There were tears of joy all around.

I was allotted a nearby apartment and given money for furniture and cooking utensils. In three days, Mubasher started at a local school, and in three weeks, I had found a job in a bank specializing in mortgages. Shaqil was placed in a government-run day care center, and the most heart-rending task was to make an apartment key for Mubasher to let himself in after school. Amir, Gulshan's husband, would not hear of it and said that Mubasher would go to Gulshan's apartment after school to be with his cousins till I came home.

I never wrote to Salim. Mubasher kept asking about him and once wrote a childish innocent letter to him which I never mailed.

Nine months later, Gulshan called me, saying Salim was in Vancouver. He called Gulshan's home, having gotten the telephone number from the Immigration Office. Shilo gave him my location. When he appeared at the door Mubasher clung to him and Shaqil, who I thought would have forgotten him, went to him immediately. My determination to leave him melted when I saw my children's reaction. I gave in, realizing it was not just the children. I was alone and vulnerable, and here he seemed so caring, loving and attentive, like some familiar comfortable security in this changed world.

He stayed home and cared for the children while I was at work. By this time our youngest sister, Shamim, and her husband, Eqbal, were also settled in Vancouver and our families had many warm and happy times together. Salim got a job at Smithrite with Amir's help.

Shamim, a doctor, called to say she was going to New York on a conference, did I want to come? I jumped at the opportunity to meet my mother and father, Amir and Nergi and their children, who by now had moved from their Brooklyn apartment to a home in Long Island, New York.

In New York, we spent the few days reminiscing about our lost lives. The most firm forward-lookers were Ma and Bapa, who assured us we would be better off here than in Uganda. We talked of the Brooklyn apartment, which had initially served as haven to so many of our family when first displaced. I was reminded of two paintings by Amir and Nergi's friend Bella Feldman. They had given them to me to send later when they had left Uganda in 1971. I had stowed them away carefully under my mattress and in the chaos of my leaving they are still there in some forgotten bed.

Salim and I lived a roller-coaster life with each other—hating and loving in turn. Eventually Amir in New York needed a trusted and trusting assistant. This was my chance to break off and fly far away. I took it, and finally Salim and I were emotionally and legally parted. Mobasher was settled into life with a partner and Shaqil would benefit, I rationalized, by some distance from me.

Mehr-u-nisa—Mary—settled in Vancouver, where she reared her two boys. Her older, Mubasher, had ambitions to fly the skies. But it was impossibly expensive to get the flying hours he needed. He started life pumping gas and his wit allowed him to slowly climb into management positions in car dealerships. He took a leap ahead and is now teaching motor mechanics at a local school. He married a Canadian, Cindy, and they now have two boys, Braiden and Owen.

Mary worked many years in Vancouver in the same field that she worked in Uganda—the mortgage department of a bank. When Amir needed a secretary cum jack-of-all-trades in New York, she jumped at this opportunity to leave Vancouver. Besides a discontented personal life, her son Shafique was finding it difficult to stabilize himself, and she felt a little distance from him might be beneficial. She was right, and he soon settled down in the absence of a mother who always baled him out. After Amir died, her job in New York was terminated. She had to return to Vancouver and was absorbed into the giant Yamato machine owned by her sister Gulshan and her brother-in-law Amir. She is content and though separated from Salim has a cordial, even warm relationship with him.

Laila's story

Laila, the fourth of Ma's nine children, was born in 1939 in Kakira just outside Kampala. The family lived in Singida, Tanzania, so in order to complete a more organized high school education, she moved to Kampala, Uganda, to live with her Uncle Musa and his daughter Sultan. There she was treated like a daughter in their extended family. The cousins Sultan and Laila remained like sisters for life. In 1966 Laila married Aneel Korde, an attorney, and I later delivered her of Rukesh, a few days older than my Sharyn, and Larissa, named after Zhivago's love, Larissa Antipova. They were well settled and content in Kampala, Aneel in a private law practice with his father in Kampala, and Laila in a secretarial situation in

*the Department of Obstetrics and Gynecology at the Makerere Medical
School and later in the British American Tobacco Company. Like us, they
considered themselves Ugandan.*

*Laila was the last of the sisters to give me her story. At first she
refused, saying it was too painful to relive. When I eventually received it,
I understood her pain. All the important people in the story, her husband,
Aneel, his father and mother, her parents and Amir, her brother and my
husband, have left us.*

This is Laila's story of those ninety days.

The date was August 8th, 1972. We were celebrating the wedding
of Suneel, Aneel's younger brother, at Nakawa College, just
outside Kampala, where his Canadian bride, Lynn, taught. Indian
and Western food and wine flowed in 'Korde style.' People were
ignoring the scattered tables and chairs and chatting in small
groups on that fateful soft Kampala evening. For a reason I cannot
remember, possibly the result of a rumor, someone switched on a
radio. Like a magnet all the guests were drawn to what was being
broadcast. Idi Amin's unmistakable voice announced that he was
giving Uganda Asians three months to get out, leave, go back where
they came from. Laughter spread amongst the group. We could not
take this seriously. Our defiance made us laugh. Remember, we
were Ugandan and third-generation Africans—although fatefully
brown.

Aneel's father made the first move toward recognition that the
threat was serious. He directed the newlyweds Suneel and Lynn
to take their newly purchased Toyota to Nairobi, Kenya, for their
honeymoon and leave it there with his sister Neela, rather than go
by train as they had planned. This was 'no joke, no mistake,' he
said. 'We have to start securing all we possess.'

And the next day proved him right.

What was to be the fate of Asians who had taken on Ugandan
citizenship? Surely this act of trust would exempt them from this
banishment edict. Amin declared that their validity was questioned,
and they had to have their papers reviewed and verified. Long
queues with people even waiting for days formed at the Uganda
Immigration Office. We had to establish our own validity and that
of Aneel's parents.

The Uganda Immigration office was looking for reasons to reject us. They declared that I had been three days late in renouncing my British citizenship and I had to revert to 'being British.' The rest of my family, they declared, were real Ugandans. Now what—did they expect me to leave without them?

August flew away. It was now September 1972. We could not accept the idea of leaving and tried to maintain a semblance of normality. Aneel was a master chess and bridge player. One evening he was playing bridge at the Goan Club. A group of soldiers burst in and demanded to know what was going on. Everyone froze. Aneel, the attorney, decided to be his friends' advocate and informed the soldiers that this was a game of bridge. The lead soldier said he was lying and it looked like gambling to him. Although as far as all knew gambling was not against the law, Aneel explained that there was no money involved. The soldier then called him 'Wahinidi.' Although *wahindi* merely means 'Indian,' when said in this manner it is accusatory and derogatory—'*Wahindi, ingiya motoca*'—'Get into the car.' Several 'disappearances' had recently occurred in just this manner, including that of a well-known attorney, Anil Clerk, who was taken from his home in the presence of his mother and was never seen again.

Aneel got into the car and was wedged into the back seat between two soldiers, one of whom pointed a gun at him. At first they drove around town without any apparent destination. They asked Aneel his line of work. When he said he was a lawyer they asked where his office was. They drove to his office on Allidina Visram Street and asked for the keys to the office, which he did not have. After some discussion they got out of the car and said, '*Toka wahindi, toka, toka*'—'Get out, Indian, get out, get out.' Aneel got out and, very cool, and walked homeward. Once the car was out of sight he started running. He ran the two miles and arrived breathless at our place. We made a firm decision to leave at that moment.

At just this time the Canadian government had announced that they would admit into Canada all Ugandan Asians who met certain criteria. They were not interested in professionals, but in blue-collar workers. A Canadian woman who played bridge with Aneel said she could get us an interview based on my being a secretary. I was employed at the British American Tobacco Company, and my boss obtained a letter from the Canadian branch of the company stating that they would be willing to offer me a job if we moved to Canada. The interview went well and we were issued a visa.

In those troubled times things seemed to be falling into place. The newlyweds Suneel and Lynn moved without a problem to Toronto, which was Lynn's home. My mother and father had been successfully sponsored by Amir and Nergesh in New York and were to leave shortly.

Aneel's parents, Baba and Mummy, decided they would go to India, where Baba had his brothers and other family. The Indian Embassy had organized a bus to take passengers from the embassy to Entebbe Airport, so on the day they were to leave, we accompanied them to the embassy. Baba embraced Aneel as he wept. It was the last time he was to see his son. Ogutu, the driver, turned away so we could not see his tears. Baba regained his composure and made Ogutu face him. He said to him, 'I will send for you when I am settled. I will need someone to drive me around. In the meantime, I have asked Aneel to transfer the car to you. Use it to taxi people around till I send for you.' All of us, and certainly Ogutu, knew he would never leave Africa, but the plan eased the moment.

Through his tears Ogutu thanked Baba, '*Asante sana, Bwana mkuba.*' Swahili words naturally change meaning according to who is being addressed, who said them and how they are said. '*Bwana mkuba*'—'great boss'—is usually used ironically about former masters or an inflated ego. Here it was used with deep respect for a kindly, elderly gentleman.

I think of Baba so often. When I was in hospital having just had my babies he would bring me chicken soup in a thermos and chicken livers fried in butter to make my blood strong again. He used to make *shira*, a sweet with a cream-of-wheat base loaded with pistachio nuts and almonds for Rukesh and Larissa, food for their developing little brains, he said. And now Rukesh, my son, makes the same *shira* for his own son with Baba's recipe.

We never saw Baba again. He died soon after he tried to start a new life in India. After his death we were fortunate to have Mummy come and live with us for many years in Toronto and then Vancouver.

In the third week of October, we took Ma and Bapa to Entebbe Airport. We passed several military checkposts, at each of which money changed hands before we were allowed on. Finally they were ready to board the aircraft, my mother leaving the land of her birth and my father leaving all his adult life behind. If these thoughts crossed their minds they never expressed them. Both were the ultimate pragmatists. We felt elated because they were going into a safe haven with Amir and Nergesh in New York, and we would meet them very soon.

Inexplicably, I forgot to let Amir and Nergesh know the particulars of their departure. Bapa said he would send a telegram, but if he did they never received it and so were not at Kennedy Airport in N.Y. to receive them. The thought of them landing alone at that vast airport with no one to greet them is unbearable. But resourceful as always, Bapa got a taxi and showed the driver Amir's address in Brooklyn. Bapa confessed before the ride that he did not have cash but that his son would pay him at the other end. The taxi driver belied the image of the surly New York cabbie and kindly accepted to take them to Brooklyn. At the other end, Amir and Nergesh were out, but little Rushna, their oldest daughter, greeted them and ran to a neighbor to borrow the fare to pay the taxi driver.

Our November 8th deadline was fast approaching, but things were working out. Our charges, all four of our parents, were out of the country. Our Canadian friends Victor and Ruth Ann offered to take any belongings to their home in Toronto. I packed photographs, jewelry and other things that, retrospectively, I could have done without, but at the time I wanted to hang onto something…anything. Other friends took money for us and repaid us in the U.S. There was not too much else we could do.

I had sold the children's outdoor slide, swing and sandbox. The buyer arrived one morning with a check for 300 shillings and proceeded to dismantle and remove the playthings. Four-year-old Rukesh climbed on the slide and refused to get down. I berated him and he cried. This was his domain being destroyed and removed, and his mother stood by and helped. I did not have the good sense to tell the man to come after we had left. I was so consumed with making a tidy departure.

It was October 30th, the day we were to leave. Early that morning the four of us gathered with Manjeri and Teresa, the ayah and help, in the living room to say our goodbyes. Aneel gave each of them 1000 shillings, a year's wages. Teresa sobbed and was barely able to blurt out, *'Kwaheri muthu yangu,'* — 'Goodbye, my people.' The dignified Manjeri said, *'Chunga watoto yangu,'* 'Look after OUR children.' In the sweetness of African culture, children are never yours or mine, but ours. When I see Rukesh and Larissa struggling with child-care problems in the U.S., I remember those two loving women. Many said Asians were punished for their derogatory attitudes toward Africans, but I believe we lived symbiotically.

Our trusted Ogutu dropped us off at the Canadian Consulate on Kampala Road. Aneel gave him the car keys and the deed to the car. *"Asante sana, Bwana dogo,"* he said. *"Si sana,"* which was the gracious way to acknowledge such heartfelt thanks, the equivalent of 'My pleasure,' but literally meaning 'Not so much.'

We climbed into the bus which was to 'safe passage' us to Entebbe Airport. We had embassy cars escorting us and were waived through the many checkpoints.

At the airport I was asked by a female security guard if I was carrying any money. I said I was not and was subject to a humiliating strip search by her. If I had money, I could have just given her the useless currency and been spared this last humiliation as I left the country of my birth.

We were finally on the plane. After the weeks of turmoil, the sudden quiet was unnerving. I remember a smooth takeoff. Larissa cried herself to sleep on my lap. She was upset because I told her I had left her pacifier at home—I thought this was a good way to rid her of the habit. Now I think upon the cruelty of this torment in addition to the child losing all that was routine and comforting in her daily life.

From my window seat I looked down on a lovely clear day at the city of green hills in the sun. The Aga Khan Mosque, the majestic building dominating old Kampala where I spent so much of my teenage life, Kololo Hill where Aneel and I went a-courting and watched the sunset and night come on with a thousand twinkling lights. I was leaving the loveliest mildest climate, always 65 to 70 degrees because even though the equator passed through the country (through a town called Equator) it was at an elevation of

3000 feet. When it rained, it poured, and afterward butterflies came out to play amongst rainbows. Our lives seemed simple compared to life in North America, sunny days and cool nights scented with jasmine and frangipani.

Kampala was receding and the pilot's voice addressed us, 'Relax, people, we have just left Ugandan soil and with it the guns, the fear, the military.' And the country of our birth. Champagne corks popped and I readied myself for a new chapter with a flute of champagne.

I am writing this in November of 2004. Bush has just won four more years and, as we are repeatedly reminded, this time with a mandate. Thirty-two years ago I was thirty-two years old and suddenly stateless as a result of a tyrant from the bush. Thirty-two years later I feel disenfranchised by another Bush-man in a country that I have ceased to understand. But this time there is no Aneel by my side to rationalize my life.

Laila and Aneel settled in Toronto, Vancouver, and finally New York. Rukesh, their son, born a few days before my youngest daughter Sharyn and delivered by me, initially did graduate work in Philosophy but then redirected and went to law school like his father. He is presently in a corporate law firm in Washington, DC, and on his way to partnership. He married Sara Werner, a Shakespearean scholar, and they have two sons, Anil and Jacob.

Larissa, their daughter, named after Zhivago's love, Larissa Antipova, became a doctor and sub-specialized in hematology/oncology. She took her fellowship training at the National Institutes of Health and is sliding comfortably into an academic, research position. She married Scott Cole, who was briefly a student clerk with me at the New York Medical College and then did an Ob/Gyn residency in Washington, DC. They have a daughter, Maya. Both families live just outside Washington, minutes away from each other.

By the time Rukesh and Larissa went to graduate school, Anil had died and Laila, a legal secretary, found ways to guide her children through expensive and arduous studies to success and settled lives after all the roaming.

Sultan's story

Shahsultan, the sixth of the nine sibs and the fourth of the girls, was born in 1943, also in Singida. From an early age, she suffered health problems that gave her a special place in the hearts of her father and her oldest brother Amir. Her seizure disorder started when she was ten years old, and Amir told me that when he went back on vacation from his studies in Bombay, he would sleep in the same bed with her as she was terrified of a seizure coming on when she was alone at night. She has been seizure-free for many years now and presently lives in Toronto. At the time of the expulsion order she was married to Lutaf, who owned a sporting goods store, and had two children, Shekufe and a baby, Aarif. This is her story of those fateful ninety days and the aftermath.

We were celebrating my daughter Shakufe's fourth birthday when we heard the news. We were stunned but saw the party to its end with a sense of unreality. There were some African guests who expressed their shock and sadness...and then left. Everyone had to look out for him or herself.

Although we were Ugandans, we were told that our passports would require verification. Lutaf waited a day and a night on line before his citizenship was affirmed. When my turn came, I was told that because I had not cancelled my British citizenship after becoming Ugandan, my Ugandan citizenship was revoked. I now had to go to the British immigration office to reestablish British citizenship.

If I had thought the experience at the Ugandan offices was bad, thE British immigration office was brutal. There were longer lines, and the office was open for only a limited number of hours during the day. The plight of the Asians did not move the British to extend us any extra help. I waited in line all of one day and then went back the next day. On the second day at lunchtime I was tired and went home to get a bite. When I returned I was admonished for leaving and expecting to retain my standing in the line. I lost my cool and raised my voice saying, 'You think we are not human because we are brown. Don't you think we, too, have needs—to drink and eat and use the bathroom?' I made such a disturbance that I was taken inside to keep me quiet. Once inside, the cold and impassive British clerk said that I did not qualify for British citizenship. I had already consulted Laila's husband, Aneel, a lawyer, who had told me that I did on the basis of my mother's British citizenship at the time of my birth. I therefore stuck to my contention and they eventually, reluctantly, agreed to issue me a British passport. I asked for my children to be put on the passport. They did so but said that at the end of a year their names should be removed. I could not argue any more and left with this arrangement.

In spite of my British passport, Lutaf and I did not want to go to England. When the Canadians opened a temporary immigration center to process the banished Asians, we applied and were readily accepted and given a date for travel.

My sister Gulshan gave us the address of a friend in Canada where our possessions could be shipped. We packed what we could, and I still have the good china that my sisters had given me as a wedding present and old photograph albums which are irreplaceable.

Lutaf and his brother tried to get some money out of the country, paying our contact locally with a promise to be paid when we reached Canada. We only recovered part of our money and never saw the rest.

We were amongst the first of our family to leave. Even when we were on the plane to Canada, we had not decided where we were headed. I worked for Gailey and Roberts in Uganda and had found a branch in Charlottetown, Prince Edward Island, but had been warned that this was a remote and difficult place to live in. Lutaf thought we should go to Edmonton to avoid the mass Asian exodus to Vancouver. While in the air, Canadian immigration officers were talking to us and suggested that Montreal would be a better choice because of more clement weather and better opportunities. The only drawback was we would have to learn French, which we felt would be an enjoyable challenge.

So with this in-flight decision Montreal it was, and we arrived at Mirabel Airport to be greeted by a host of welcoming volunteers. Aarif was only ten months old and was whisked away to have his diaper changed. We were taken into a large hall where we chose coats, sweaters, boots and scarves from piles of donated clothing. After a hot dinner we were taken to the YMCA where we were made comfortable. They even had a crib for Aarif. The next day they instructed us on how to obtain social insurance cards and how to go about looking for a job. Shakufe started in a local kindergarten and I had day-care assistance for Aarif.

A few days later Lutaf's mother, brother Anu and his wife joined us at the YMCA. They brought us news of the whereabouts of the rest of the family. And I learnt that my sisters Gulshan, Mary and Shamim had made it safely to Vancouver.

We stayed two months at the YMCA. We had not yet secured jobs, but the Canadians gave us some money to rent an apartment. Our family and Lutaf's brother's family with their mother rented a three-bedroom apartment in Longueil, a suburb of Montreal. The Canadians were astoundingly and persistently kind. Many families invited us over for the day to familiarize us with the Canadian way of life. They also organized day trips for us. One took us to an ashram in the Laurentian Mountains. Lutaf was given tickets to go to an ice hockey game and as a result became a life-long fan of the sport.

We enrolled for French classes. We had three teachers. One was a Frenchman who knew no English. The second was a native Indian who hardly ever came to class. The third was an Englishman who was very keen on learning Swahili, which we happily obliged with. So we did not get to learn much French.

Lutaf found a job working in a sporting goods store with a salary of $90 a week. It wasn't much but was a start. One of his colleagues was specially kind and often invited us to his home and made the children and me feel very welcome. I found it hard to get a permanent placement and through an agency did a number of temporary secretarial jobs. This helped but I really had to work on my French.

Lutaf's brother and his family and mother moved to an independent apartment. This made things more difficult for us financially and I lost the services of Ma (Lutaf's mother) to look after the children, but I found a babysitter and she turned out to be a real darling. She entered our lives from nowhere and seemed to immediately and unconditionally love our children—never seemed to want to leave at the end of the day and tarried on with affectionate goodbyes—and would never accept more money than what was agreed upon. The word 'refugees' brought tears to her eyes.

By this time, my sister Laila had settled in Toronto. I applied for and got a job there. Laila and her family moved to another apartment, and we moved into the one they had been renting. She helped me placing Shakufe in school and finding a babysitter for Aarif.

We were slowly establishing a life in Canada. It was a struggle but our hard work has paid off. I found a stable and pleasant secretarial position and Lutaf found the work he knew best, in a sport's goods store. Although he did not own it as he did in Uganda, it allowed him to work close to his love of all games and sports.

Sultan moved from Montreal to Toronto and has been there ever since. Several years into her marriage, she followed her heart and left her husband to move in with Arnold, a caring, loving, attentive retiree. She was the love and the all of his life and she blossomed into a vocal politically and artistically aware person. Five years later Arnold developed aplastic anemia and gradually weakened. We went to give her support at his funeral and were happy to see the person who had taken charge of the arrangements was the ever-faithful Lutaf. And, to end this story on an upbeat note, they are now reconciled and together again.

Sultan's daughter, Shakufe ('blossom' in Persian), whom I had delivered in 1968, became a physiotherapist and later took an accounting qualification. Her son, Aarif, is a lawyer in Toronto. Both were married in 2006

Shamim's story

Delivered by an Indian lay midwife at home in 1949 in Singida, Tanzania, Shamim was the eighth of the nine sibs and the youngest of the five sisters. In this large family, she often felt overlooked and called herself 'nani ne sareli'—small and rotten. But she alone amongst the girls went on to college and medical school and, years later in Canada, while practicing as a radiologist, also earned her credentials as a lawyer.

When Amin signed the expulsion order, Shamim had recently qualified as a doctor from Makerere Medical School in Kampala and married Eqbal Bhimji, her high school sweetheart. After her wedding and a European/

*Canadian honeymoon, they settled in Fort Portal in southwest Uganda,
close to the Congo border where Eqbal and his family owned several
businesses and had tea estates. They were in Fort Portal when they heard
the expulsion order. This is her story of the 90 days.*

I had never had the need to own a passport. In 1971, when Bapa
was obtaining a passport for my brother Pheroze to go to England,
he arranged for mine as well. I therefore acquired a Ugandan
passport by serendipity. As a matter of pride, Bapa had made
clear on the passport that I was a doctor. In the chaotic days that
followed Amin's expulsion order, this chance fact had the potential
of causing unforeseen problems.

After we were married, Eqbal and I traveled over Europe and
Canada. While in Canada (this is prior to the Amin edict) we looked
into the possibility of emigrating to Canada. They were happy to
have us, but we would have to stay in Canada for three months to
have the process finalized. Since I was in the middle of an internship
and Eqbal had business commitments, we decided to take the
application forms and apply at our leisure via Beirut, which was
the center through which African applications were processed.

When we returned to Uganda, we found that Idi Amin had
already started making difficulties for the Asians, requiring all
of them to carry a *kipande*—a red identification card similar to
passbooks that were carried by blacks in South Africa when in
'white territory' after dark. Since Bapa and one of Eqbal's cousins
had put in applications for us while we were still out of the country,
we acquired these humiliating documents painlessly. Most of the
other Asians spent days in line to obtain them. Seething, we kept
saying to ourselves, 'We were born here like all you blacks. Our
mother was born here.' My passbook was dated February, 1972.

I finished my internship at Mulago Hospital in Kampala and
moved to Fort Portal to work as a junior surgical officer. The senior
surgeon, a Britisher, developed jaundice soon after I arrived and
was taken to Kampala, where he was found to have a hepatoma
from which he died soon after. So in spite of my inexperience, I was
the only surgeon working with an obstetrician, an internist and two
other junior officers at the Buhinga Government Hospital, the only
general hospital in Fort Portal.

It was at this time that Amin had his divine dream and announced that Asians were given 90 days to leave the country. That evening, when we were home from work, we discussed the situation and decided to leave Fort Portal for Kampala and work out arrangements to leave the country.

Within the week I resigned my position, and Eqbal had wound up what he could, packed a couple of bags and drove the 200 miles to Kampala. We had difficulty finding a place to stay as Ma and Bapa had a tiny apartment and all my brothers were out of the country. My sisters were in Kampala, but were immersed in their own problems. We stayed at Kitante at the home of Eqbal's sister's boyfriend, who was a teacher at Kitante Primary School. His home was provided by his employer, the Uganda government.

Since we had recently visited Vancouver and liked the place, this is where we decided to go. Although Canada did not have a presence in Uganda, within a few days they had set up temporary headquarters in the basement of the Kampala Public Library to process potential immigrants and refugees. When we presented our papers, which we had intended to send via Beirut with a provisional acceptance from the Canadian Government, we were quickly processed, and I believe we may have been the first Asian couple to receive our papers with instructions that we could leave for Canada at any time.

We were not in any rush. The thought 'Did we really have to go?' nagged us. In any case, Eqbal wanted to stay as long as feasible to attend to his various businesses.

I found time on my hands and volunteered to work at the Canadian consulate to help process the medical examinations required for the Asian applicants. I spent a lot of time drawing blood, examining urine and stools. 'Senior' doctors did the physical examination, but because of this job I was able to expedite the process for my sisters Sultan and Gulshan and Eqbal's sister's boyfriend, whose place we were staying at. Aneel, my sister Laila's husband, was a prominent lawyer in the city and was making the arrangements for his family, his parents and Ma and Bapa. Aneel was a cool and quiet operator, and with the help of strategic bribes, was able to look after much of the family. Mary (Nisa) had decided not to leave since she was married to an African. (*See Nisa's story.*)

When I was not working I was busy shopping. I guess I wanted to maintain the semblance of normality. I bought cutlery, dishes, *godras* (handmade softest comforters), tape decks, clothes—all the material things that seemed so important at the time. I went to Drapers, the only department store in Kampala, and chose a china set with a red flower and green leaf pattern, almost all of which is now broken or lost. I was getting these wrapped and packed when Eqbal came rushing into Drapers, telling me to drop everything and come with him.

When we exited on Kampala Road there were people and cars fleeing from the center of town. The rumor was that the Tanzanians had invaded in support of Obote, the deposed prime minister, who had been given refuge by his friend Julius Nyerere in Tanzania. The helicopters were said to have landed near the high courts and the streets were being evacuated. We left my car at Drapers and drove off in Eqbal's car. The road to Kitante where we were staying was packed. Many had abandoned their cars and were fleeing on foot. We turned toward Ma's house in old Kampala and finally reached there and waited till things quieted. We learnt later what had actually happened. The Chief Justice of Uganda, Benedicto Kiwanuka, had been dragged out of the courthouse where he was presiding—to his ultimate death. A feeling of unreality precluded all else—anger, fear, loss and sadness.

We did not want to 'wait and see what happened' any longer and decided to purchase our airline tickets. The nagging thought remained, that we were Uganda citizens and initially Uganda citizens were not required to leave. We also had college loans to pay back and I had pledged to work in Government hospitals for two years (I had only worked eight months). Additionally, Amin had said that doctors were required not to leave the country out of patriotic considerations, and Bapa had made quite sure that the fact that I was a doctor was clearly written on my passport.

All these thoughts were clouding our minds. As a means to use as much money as possible, we decided to buy tickets for a three-month world tour. Toward this, Eqbal had withdrawn a large amount of cash for the purchase. The tickets and remaining cash were in a safe in his offices at Nyanza Motors on Allidina Visram Street where his cousin Bashir was a business partner.

Word apparently got out that there was a large amount of foreign currency in this office, and a truckload of soldiers arrived at the office to search the premises. They found the safe and made Bashir open it to reveal the world tour airline tickets and 30,000 Uganda shillings.

A sad commentary of this anxious time was how it pitted victim against victim, family members against each other. Bashir, unasked, declared the money to be Eqbal's. Eqbal said the money was for more airline tickets, and in any case the currency was local and not foreign. The soldiers demanded to be taken to Bashir's home to continue their search. Bashir's wife Mumtaz and I were just preparing to leave the house (more purchases) when they arrived. Bashir told his wife in Gujerati that they were looking for foreign currency and petrified Mumtaz said 'Mari pase che'—'I have some.' It turned out that she had a small amount of Zaire money, which did not interest them. They were looking for U.S. dollars or British pounds. We were furious with Bashir—but there was more treachery to come from him.

We confirmed our airline tickets to London to visit Eqbal's parents and then go on to Vancouver. Now that we were clearly leaving, I wanted to return to Fort Portal to pack our belongings, including jewelry, photographs and other things I thought were invaluable. Eqbal thought it was unsafe and crazy to return to Fort Portal. We had recently heard of our friend Zuli, who had been taken away from his home in Fort Portal for 'questioning.' A ransom was demanded for his return, which his wealthy family paid. The day after his release, the family went to the mosque to offer thankful prayers for his release. Zuli said he would stay home to bathe and rest. When the family returned home, they found he had committed suicide. It was rumored he could not handle the things that were done to him while in custody.

Over Eqbal's objections I left for Fort Portal with a driver.

I assembled a number of tea chests, of which there was an abundance on our tea plantations. I packed about 25 of these chests with my belongings. As each chest was filled I moved it to the verandah to prepare it for loading onto a truck that would transport them to Kampala. Eqbal's cousin Shabir came to help me. Suddenly a young black man was in the circular driveway demanding to know what we were up to. We explained that we were packing in preparation to leave the country. An argument ensued with the man saying we had no right to take things out of the country as everything now belonged to the state. Things got heated and ugly, and I told Shabir in Gujerati that I had a gun in the house and I was going to get it. Eqbal always carried a handgun when he went to the estates to pay the workers. He started this practice after one of his partners was robbed while paying weekly wages to the tea plantation workers. However, I could not find the gun and later learned that Eqbal had rounded up all the arms he had — revolvers, hand-guns, rifles and B-B guns — and thrown them in the local Panga River so as not to be in possession of a weapon in these uncertain times.

I did not need the gun as a lot of back and forth yelling eventually caused the man to leave. As I was done with the packing, I called the office to send the truck down to be loaded. The truck arrived ten minutes later with an African driver and an Asian employee and relative of Eqbal's called Fida. Fida's mother had been adopted by Eqbal's grandmother. The men started loading the truck. Suddenly several army trucks entered the driveway, led by the man who had threatened us earlier. Our truck was now surrounded by army vehicles and personnel. The soldiers ordered us to line up and started their questioning. Fida said he had nothing to do with this scene and was about to walk off, but was ordered back into the lineup. Fida tried several times to distance himself from 'this Bhimji business,' and he was finally ordered into the back of the truck.

Shabir started to object and was cuffed over the head and also ordered into the back of the truck. One of the soldiers grabbed my hair and started pulling me toward the truck, when another of them said 'Wacha yeye' — 'Leave her.' It turned out that I had treated his mother at Buhinga Hospital. They waved me into the house and loaded the rest of the tea chests onto the truck. Several of them climbed into the truck and ordered the driver to follow the rest of the army vehicles, leaving me alone in the house.

I tried to call Eqbal but found that the telephone lines were dead. I ran out into the street and knocked at a neighbor's door with no response. I tried several other houses, too, but no one would open the door because word had spread that the army had come to my house. No one wanted to get involved.

I ran down the street to Eqbal's office—a hard twenty-minute run. I tried unsuccessfully to reach him, but managed to get Bapa in Kampala and told him to find Eqbal urgently. Bapa found a friend to drive him to Eqbal's office in Nyanza Motors. Finally Eqbal called me and I explained the situation. He told me to stay put, that he would get back to me.

Eqbal called Ali, a friend and an adjutant in the army with whom he had socialized in Fort Portal. He told him what had happened and asked for help. As it happened Ali had been leaving for Kampala from Fort Portal and had seen the Bhimjis Ltd. truck in army possession. He had stopped the convoy to ask what was going on. They said their orders were not to allow any tea chests to be removed as Indians were using them to smuggling gold out of the country. He told them to take the truck to the police station and not the army headquarters as this was a criminal matter. Luckily they agreed, and Ali went back to his office to sort the matter out when he received Eqbal's call. Ali suggested I spend the night with relatives and go to the police station in the morning. Ali would be there and the chests opened in his and my presence.

Meanwhile Shabir, Fida and the driver were put into a jail cell. Their belts, shoelaces and wallets were taken from them, and they spent the night on the cold floor. At 6 am, I took a thermos of tea and some food to them. The chests were opened and since nothing more significant than household goods was found, he ordered the officer to send the truck to Kampala with an army escort to be delivered to 'the people from Bhimjis Ltd.' Shabir and I went home, showered and drove to Kampala at breakneck speed.

A couple of days later, Eqbal was told to come to Wandegaya to pick up the truck. When he went there the officer demanded money in exchange. Eqbal attemped to talk to him but he said threateningly, 'Sasa wwe ne jewuna, eh?' —'Are you going to start an argument?' Eqbal handed over whatever cash he had—about 400 Uganda shillings—and drove the truck back to his office at Nyanza Motors. We added my purchases from Kampala and sent the chests to Vancouver via Mombasa with many bribes to ease the way. We never expected to see the chests again, but three months later they arrived in Vancouver. The only mishap was that a can of tumeric had leaked and my precious godra reeked of spices and was stained bright yellow. The rest of the things were enjoyed by us for years after, all the sweeter because of the cost we had been put through.

From Fort Portal I had also collected my jewelry and that belonging to Eqbal's mother and sister. There were constant tales of Asians on the way to Entebbe Airport being stopped and strip-searched and often having 'huge hoards' of jewelry confiscated from their person. Of course, to the typically Indian woman, jewelry is much more than adornment. It is her money in the bank—her insurance against adversity, a faithless husband. When she marries, all her possessions are jointly possessed by her and her husband, but her jewelry, particularly her gold, is her own.

I gave my cache of jewelry to some friends who were priests at our mosque, telling them if they ever could get the stuff out of the country we would appreciate it—otherwise to put it to any worthy use. Six years later, one of these friends brought it to London and tried to contact Eqbal's parents who had long before emigrated to Canada. Not daunted, they went through the London phone book and found a Bhimji who was Eqbal's aunt and owned some of the jewelry. Four years later when she came to Canada she brought it with her, so that ten years later it found its way to me. And then, a few years after that, our home in Vancouver was broken into and all of it finally and permanently disappeared.

As the time to leave drew closer, we were deciding what to pack in the two suitcases we were allowed. My sister Sultan's husband Lutaf owned a sporting goods store and was selling as much as he could preparatory to leaving the next day. We decided to buy tennis and badminton rackets. As we were leaving our office at Nyanza Motors we had yet another brush with the army. Two armed soldiers, an officer and two civilians, made us get out of the car and forced us back into the office where stood the same treacherous Bashir who had broken faith with us once before. The group produced a piece of paper on which was written Akbar Bhimji, who they said they were looking for. As before, Bashir pointed to Eqbal and told them that this was their man. They ordered Eqbal to come with them for questioning.

Eqbal was amazingly calm and managed to get from them what the offense was supposed to have been. It turned out that this man Akbar Bhimji (who was Bashir's brother) had driven down from

Fort Portal in Eqbal's car ten days ago. Eqbal said he had left Fort Portal three months ago and Ali, the man who had previously helped, could corroborate. A call was put through to Ali, but the phones being what they were, the call would not go through till three hours later. The civilian amongst them kept goading them to leave with Eqbal, but the name Ali apparently was powerful enough to prevent the officer from so doing. Eventually, the five of them left, saying they would be back to receive the call. Like perfect and trusting fools we waited for them. Eventually Ali called and we related our problem to him. He confirmed and said he would vouch for Eqbal's story. He stayed on the line for the next six hours waiting for the group to return but they never did. Eventually he advised us not to go back home but to spend the night elsewhere.

Our bags were in the car and we unbelievably decided — against all good judgment — to purchase our sports goods anyway. While in Lutaf's store we ran into my oldest sister, Gulshan, who, with her husband, Amir, and three children, had moved into the Apollo Hotel since their home on Mbuya hill was too remote for safety. She asked us to join them for a last 'celebratory' dinner at the hotel restaurant. After this, we checked into the hotel and spent our last night in Uganda in comfort.

The next morning we boarded a bus with armed security guards. We left our car on the street with keys in the ignition, so anyone who wished to use it would not have to break in.

Security at the airport was tight, and to my relief no one paid any attention to my being a doctor and therefore asking me not to leave. A body-search and a bribe later, we boarded the plane. When the plane took off a cheer arose from the passengers but it was not till the pilot announced, 'Ladies and gentlemen we have cleared Uganda air space,' that we clapped, hugged and literally danced in the aisles. Some anxiety recurred when we stopped for refueling at Benghazi and armed Libyan soldiers boarded the plane. Khaddafi was a good friend of Amin — could they have connected? But they left and the plane took off for London, where we were to spend a few days with Eqbal's parents before we left for Canada.

At Heathrow Airport we were herded animal-like to Immigration. The immigration officer, a woman, was contemptuous and rude.

'I suppose you have come to live in this country,' said she.

'No, we are visiting family and then going to Canada.'

'That's what they all say,' she said.

We showed her our airline tickets to Vancouver, but she remained skeptical and over our objections stamped entry for three months. We argued to make it two weeks—a question of pride and anger at her innuendos. She stamped the three months anyway.

We visited with Eqbal's parents for two weeks, and the eternally treacherous cousin Bashir, who had sold us out twice, was also there. This was no time for recriminations.

We arrived in Montreal on October 30th, 1972, and flew on to Vancouver the same day. Canada welcomed us with smiles and warmth. A Canadian volunteer group met us, swathed us in warm jackets and drove us to the Buchanan Hotel in downtown Vancouver. They almost lovingly told us to settle in and report to the Immigration Office when we were up to it.

Two days later we were walking down Robson Street, and I heard an old familiar voice: 'Shamim.' We turned around and saw Gulshan and Amir. We hugged and laughed and wept right there on the street. Halfway around the world into the unknown and you meet your sister walking down the street.

The Asian exodus from Uganda brought Shamim and her husband Eqbal to Vancouver, and they have been there since. Having completed her medical studies at Makerere Medical School in Kampala, she trained in radiology and has practiced as a radiologist since. Not satisfied with this, she went to part-time law school and graduated as a lawyer in 2002. Her special project and thesis was on Sharia Law—the law of Islam.

Her daughter, Chantal and son, Omar, went to McGill University in Montreal. Chantal is presently finding herself and Omar is busy making the world a cleaner, better place to live in.

TEN

Bookend

At the end of it all, I have lived the longest stretch of my life in the U.S. Twenty-six years in India, eleven in Uganda and the remaining in this country. 'Where is your home?' people often ask. Nothing, nowhere. But the sun-dappled East African parks with wild wild fauna do flash in and out.

What makes home? The birth of one's children—so it may be Africa. The death of one's dearest. So it is right here in the States. Amir died suddenly while we were on holiday in Mumbai for the fiftieth-year reunion of our medical school class. He died unexpectedly in the quiet, in the early hours of deep night in my sister's home in Mumbai. In the very apartment where we had been married. Others saw some pattern and reason to this. I saw nothing. There followed unspeakable hours. Calls to our daughters, unsuspecting innocents, pleased to hear my voice till they heard what I had to tell them. A surreal trip home with him flying somewhere in the cargo carriage of the plane and me in a window seat. Flying above the clouds for a last voyage together. We buried him days later. This will eventually bind me to this country. One day I will say 'Home? Right here.'

I remember thinking when I first started practice in Uganda, that I would eventually give up the irregularity of obstetrics and just practice gynecology—scheduled office work and surgery practice with little emergency. There is no specialty other than obstetrics where each patient's story ends in an unpredictable emergency. Unpredictable in time and often unpredictable in outcome. How could one adjust a life to inevitable unpredictables?

But the exact opposite transpired. The fetus, hidden patient, captured my fancy, and the woman who generously housed it became my muse.

While I was completing my residency in the U.S., the subspecialty of maternal-fetal medicine (MFM) was being legitimized. In 1973, after completing residency at the Methodist Hospital in Brooklyn, I was accepted into an MFM fellowship at the Nassau County Medical Center in East Meadow, Long Island, New York. Dr. Leon Mann, my fellowship director, had been allotted two positions. My co-fellow was Dr. Amrutha Bhaktavatsalan. She did not mind being called 'Ruth,' extracted from the depths of her first name. She would be the 'animal lab' fellow and I the 'clinical.'

My work was mundane compared to the glamour and precision of the sheep lab. There the staff formed a close and collegial group with Leon Mann heading the exploration into the mysteries of placental transfer and fetal brain function. The pregnant ewe was their experimental animal. An astoundingly placid animal, who tolerated all manner of indignity. Electrodes and sampling tubes implanted in multiple sites, all coming out of the ovine's side into a 'pocket.' Every aspect of the sheep was being invaded and monitored, and it would be quietly, sheepishly chewing its cud. Amongst the last experiments done in that lab was the study of the effects of fetal thyroidectomy--intricate surgery involving delivering the sheep fetus, removing its thyroid gland and returning it to the ewe's uterus to continue the pregnancy. When term pregnancy was reached, the ewe was delivered and the fetus 'sacrificed.' Each fetal organ was studied to determine what changes absence of the thyroid gland would cause. Ruthlessness and precision in the laboratory. Unfortunately often not equivalent to the human condition.

But I did learn enormously. Although Dr. Mann did not have the stomach for emergency work, his analysis of cases and distillation of them, from whimsical 'art' to physiology and some degree of science, was a new experience. This was evidence-based teaching, even before it became a favorite buzzword. At the end of my fellowship he asked me to continue as a junior attending on the service. I remember he offered me the position one rainy evening in the hospital car park. He only had a meager salary line from a part-time physician who had left. I eagerly and happily accepted to do a major full-time job for a part-time salary.

With Dr. Mann's help we investigated and published several papers on fetal medicine. Initially the ideas were his, the legwork mine. Writing the paper in sparse precise quantitative and not qualitative terms I found most difficult of all. To remove all qualitative detail and to present the work objectively in minimal words came to me with difficulty. The seemingly simple fact that I learnt very slowly was that a medical paper has four parts. An introduction explains the reasons for performing the study. A methods section is exactly that, followed by results and a discussion. Only after years did I realize that if the first two sections were well thought out, the last two would follow easily. The results section would answer line for line what was outlined in 'methods.' It was so simple and elegant, yet it took me long to grasp this. An initial set of investigations was on the state of oxygenation of the fetus in labor, based on the technique of obtaining fetal blood from the presenting scalp. And another set was on observations of fetal growth failure. And the joy JOY! of seeing my own name in print in peer-reviewed journals.

In 1976 Dr. Mann left for another position and advised me to look around as well, as he felt the academics and the investigative atmosphere that I loved would deteriorate with his departure. I traveled to San Francisco, where I was offered a job at the San Francisco General Hospital, but Amir failed to find a position. Later in 1979, on a wild impulse, we traveled to Hawaii, where the same problem repeated.

In retrospect, I cannot imagine a childhood in Hawaii for the children. The East Coast of the U.S. in some intangible way gave us the civilization I sought even in the face of aberrant governments that were elected to office.

But the academics continued now under my guidance. I continued to direct the fellowship program Dr. Mann had started. My line of investigation was analysis of the obstetric antecedents of brain injury in the infant.

I 'acted' as chairMAN for the next few years, not wanting the job, which was eventually given to an internal candidate, the chief of the Family Planning Services, benign and quiet Dr. Joel Robbins. One of his first orders of business was to restore my disparate salary. It so happened that at that very time the then Nassau County Executive had inordinately raised the salary of some of his cronies. This was discovered, and all county employees with unusual salary increments were put on 'a list.' My name was on the list with the cronies. They eventually came to some kind of justice and I was 'unlisted.'

Dr. Robbins died a slow and painful death from pancreatic cancer and was succeeded by a Harvard academic as chairman. He was a born-and-bred Boston Brahmin, and his reason for descending into New York was never clear. He galled us by prefacing each of his pronouncements (and there were many) by what the practice at Harvard had been. And most astounding, he confided to me that he had a deep distrust of Indians and found them to be uniformly intellectually dishonest. Shades of my first encounters with colonials in Uganda. What was clear was there was not enough room for the two of us. He told me this on many occasions and I agreed.

One evening I was working late and answered a call. It was Dr. Jim Jones, the recently appointed chair at New York Medical College (NYMC), an institute 'in the Catholic tradition,' calling to see if I was interested in heading his division of Maternal-Fetal medicine. As I drove to the interview in Valhalla, NY, Wagner's 'The Gods Enter Valhalla' played all the way on NPR. I took it as a sign.

I must lack the essence of a true medical academician because I spent seventeen years at my first real position at the Nassau County Medical Center and the next eleven years at the NYMC. Restlessness, moving, shifting to crawl ever upwards was not part of my life. Of course it could have been inertia and lack of personal ambition, although ego I did not lack. I directed a Maternal Fetal medicine division and later became Director of the Obstetrics and Gynecology Department. One of the most satisfying parts of this job was running the fellowship program in Maternal-Fetal Medicine. Although I had done this in my previous position, I now trained a group of exceptional fellows who continue to excel academically, converse intellectually and have the same yen to investigate and publish as I had. This led into the end of the century.

Incumbent upon Directorship was also managing the finances of the department. And although my pathological fear of debt led the department to solvency, my joy in my work disappeared. I unceremoniously but voluntarily stepped down and was touched at the goodbyes I received. There was the inevitable clock gift. What could these retirement timepieces mean? A reminder that time moves on?

I accepted a part-time position in the clinics—and bided some time there. One day I arrived at the high-risk clinic and listened to the radio a nurse had switched on. It was the morning of 9/11/01. The clinic had a lecture theatre on the main floor with a mammoth TV screen and a group of us—doctors, nurses, housekeepers, patients, cafeteria staff, security guards—watched as the second tower was hit. With a jolt I realized that Cena, my middle daughter, by now a medical student, was in the downtown area of the city doing a rotation at New York University.

Out the window from the clinic a surreal scene was playing out. The hospital shared its campus with many institutions, one of which was the Westchester County Correctional Facility. While the towers in Manhattan were being demolished, the guards were so occupied watching what was occurring on television that a group of prisoners escaped. And out the windows of the clinic were the swat team in black jumpsuits rounding up the escapees. My children were safe and Cena stayed on at the hospital, but as everyone remembers there were many deaths but few hospital admissions. She walked back home over Brooklyn Bridge to her home in Park Slope.

The clinic job gave me little joy. The two expert nurse practitioners who were the constant features at the clinic hardly needed any help, and the residents regarded clinic as a chore to get through as fast as possible to get back to 'real' work.

Amir and I were to go to Mumbai for our fifty-year medical school reunion, and I decided to retire completely after our return. Amir traveled extensively because of the international nature of his job and I thought I would tag along and travel as old people tend to do as long as they are able. And then back to the top of this chapter.

So he died, left. It really irritates me when people think it softens the event by saying 'passed away.' In a fit of masochism I retired anyway. But a few weeks later I was offered a consultancy in the Bronx at the Jacobi Medical Center. I have been there since but have worked the job into a mainly teaching position. Part-time, and deep with those young residents whom I love second only to pregnant women.

Amir was an activist from our early and precarious days. Not many accept my knowledge that he was a pessimist—a pessimist, but daring and ambitious. In the pyramidal system at the then (now long gone) Brooklyn Jewish Hospital, he was selected as one of two chief residents. The residency was run by a dour but exacting chairman, Dr. Charlie Pryles, whose job was threatened by the administration for the supposed crime of 'trying to make it Harvard.' Punished for excellence. Amir organized a protest on behalf of the residents in support of Dr. Pryles, and forever after 'grudged' those who did not join. The protest came to naught and Dr. Pryles stepped down.

After his pediatric boards, he sub-boarded in pediatric nephrology, abbreviated to 'kids' kidneys.' And then he took off. He spent a brief time as an attending at Methodist Hospital of Brooklyn (after I had left). We always claimed that things worked well personally between us because at no time did we ever work together. This is probably true—our styles were totally different. I have read about and known couples so compatible that they spent every waking—and sleeping—hour with each other. Joan Didion in her grief expressed this when her husband, John Gregory Dunne, died as suddenly as did Amir. But I never knew this and ascribed our compatibility to the hours we spent apart, later gossiping and ranting and just plain recounting the day's events. A different kind of closeness.

Amir joined the Downstate Medical Center in Brooklyn as head of the Pediatric Nephrology division and became the darling 'Papa Smerf' of a faithful group of children whose kidneys had failed and were on dialysis or had received kidney transplants and were on lifelong immunosuppressive therapy. He used all those methods we are warned against, shameless bribery and promises, to make his children live that difficult compliant life filled with strict dietary restrictions, medications, emergencies, hours on dialysis, complicated surgeries. The occasional and inevitable death filled that whole family and ours with gloom and Amir with unending remorse and regret at what might have been done.

Soon he was involved in maintaining a national registry of children with end-stage renal disease, and this translated into multiple original studies benefiting his sick sick children with serious kidney disease. And he was a veritable Croesus where funding was concerned. Although he was not calculating in our private finances, he was wily and political with his professional funds—to his and his muse's advantage.

In his final years he got so involved in the administration of his grants and the development of national protocols and studies, that he discontinued clinical practice and moved to New York Medical College, to the delight of the research and grants office and the Pediatrics Department. It was while he was here that we took that final trip to India.

And there were other deaths. It is a difficult truth, but this country became mine after the deaths.

It was a large family assembled here in North America secondary to the Amin exodus. Amir's parents had nine children with as many spouses, their children, and as years went by, the children's children. Upwards of fifty people at celebratory events. But first the deaths.

1989: Aneel Khanderao Korde

The first to leave was Aneel, Laila's husband. A practicing lawyer in Kampala, he was required to requalify in this new life. But, like many who fled their homes where they had been established and respected, it was an indignity, practically an impossibility, to go through the process again. He found employment in a legal publishing company in Canada but finally came to New York, went through an accelerated training period and took the bar examinations. As though this were not enough, the test papers at his Center were lost and he had to take the test again—and had no difficulty passing. He at last got a job that he really enjoyed as assistant district attorney in Queens. After years of a professionally gray scene he was in his element. His marriage blossomed and all was well. And just when he seemed to have recaptured a reason for living, he suffered a major heart attack and died in being transferred to a larger facility where the procedures he needed could be performed. A yellow butterfly magnolia grows luxuriantly where his ashes are scattered.

1998: Fatima Amersey Tejani

Ma, Amir's mother, was born in the Arab-influenced coastal town of Lamu in Kenya. And though she lived her married life inland and away from the coast, she retained that Arab style. The way she cooked with coconut transforming the ordinary into the extraordinary. And the way she spoke Swahili. Very different from other Asians in Uganda whose Swahili was poisoned by Gujerati. She toned down her daily Swahili so that others could understand. But when her friend, the coastal memvuvalla—banana seller— came visiting at her back door, the two would sit down to those pure Swahili chats.

She moved from Mengo in Uganda to Sultanhamud, where she was the schoolteacher's wife, occupied in her passionate way with the economy of her house and an ever-increasing family. And then she moved to Singida as the storekeeper's wife. They then moved back to the 'big city,' Kampala, initially to a small cramped apartment—Blue Room—called after the bar they lived above, and then to Madras Gardens where I first met her.

She dealt well with leaving Uganda. When she first arrived in Brooklyn in 1972, she was entranced by the material wealth around her. She, who was a 'from scratch' cook, picked up every prepared food that caught her eye. In three months she had put on so much weight that she laughed and showed me how she could not close the 'side buttons' of her dress. While other older people who had to leave their homes in Kampala did badly and were unable to adjust—there were many deaths in the year after the expulsion— not Ma. She often told of how free she felt without the African house help that was a constant burden to her. She always felt that the help, being paid, should do the job exactly, but exactly, as she thought right. She had been a harsh mistress and was relieved not to have to deal with that anymore.

She eventually moved with her husband to a well-appointed apartment in Vancouver, close to three of her daughters, who were her constant visitors. She felt good, ate well, walked in the park and attended the mosque regularly. Her family cared for her. The Ismaili community enfolded her. And her life was full and rested, as that passionate woman deserved after a long, tumultuous journey.

In 1998 she went in for 'routine' knee replacement surgery. A frantic phone call late at night told that she had bled into the surgical area and had decompensated. She never recovered, and all the east coast Tejanis took the sad transcontinental flight to Vancouver to say goodbye.

2000: Hadibhai Noormohamed Tejani

Bapa, Amir's father, was a tall, fair, handsome, quietly charismatic person, full of stories. He was born in ancient Dholka in India. He schooled and went to Garrasia College, also in India. In late teenage he responded to an advertisement for a teaching position within the Ismaili mosque in Mengo near Kampala, Uganda. Without consultation with his family—maybe even without telling them— he got together the money and made the ocean crossing to Mombasa in the late 1920's. Soon after his arrival he met a formidable Ismaili woman at a mosque who said she had a very marriageable younger sister in Lamu, an island off the coast of East Africa. So he appeared at his future wife's doorstep. Adventurous spirit he lacked not. The matter was quickly decided and they had a simple wedding solemnized at the Lamu Ismaili mosque, and the two young people sailed to the mainland in a dhow.

After three years' teaching in Mengo, he was sent to Sultanhamud in Kenya where the Ismailis had a small community and lacked a teacher. After several years of teaching the local Asian children, including his own, he could no longer support his rapidly expanding family on a teacher's salary. The family moved to Singida in Tanganyika, where he ran a general store. Years later they moved to Kampala, where he embarked on several businesses, the last of which dealt in suitcases. His suitcase store was converted into Amir's practice space, and he, Bapa, would spend most of his day facilitating the running of the house, the running of the practice, the running of the tolerant and inclusive version of Ismaili-ism he practiced.

Amir's old pal Noordin—who had lent him the money to make the plane journey to come to Bombay and marry me—gave Bapa a job as his accountant in his last years in Kampala. This was a happy and fulfilling time for him. He had a steady salary and independence. Although he had no formal qualification, he did have the best credentials. He was honest and he could close his eyes and answer more or less any arithmetic problem. He did not make mistakes. And he was fast.

He tolerated Amin's expulsion order with characteristic calm and with Ma lived with us in New York and then in an independent apartment in Queens. He was restless, she always complained. Restless. Before anyone could complete a list of groceries, he would have vanished on the mission. When he returned and was told he had forgotten things, before hearing all that was forgotten he would be off again. But here, with just the two of them and without the tension of having to deal with children, racial tensions and house help, they slowly became friends. After all these years of strife and conflict, things were quiet and they were friends.

They moved to Vancouver to a happy independent life surrounded by family and friends. There she died. And he, who was very dependent on her, was left alone. His working daughters found a place for him in an assisted living facility. But by this time he was regressing and retreating. Quite proficient in English, he now preferred to speak only Gujerati. Quite inured to Western food, now he wanted his old comfort foods, the one that she had cooked for him from the time she was his teenaged bride in faraway Lamu, Sultanhamud, Singida and Kampala. How could he relate to bingo and bowling?

His son Pheroze and Pheroze's redheaded Irish wife, Mella, decided to make a home for him. With our help they remodeled the main floor of their comfortable home in the Poconos, Pennsylvania, and he spent his last years with them surrounded by laughing Pheroze, hearty, cheery Mella and their two teenaged children, who loved and respected him. They lightened his last years. His immediate memory appeared to be failing but he would surprise us with early Africa stories told with delicate detail.

This is the story of his last day.

He had lived ninety-two years, eleven months and some days. This was to be his last. Some time during the night he was visited. The visitor made a mark on him. An indelible mark. He called out at the time: 'Mella, Mella, is it time?'

'No, Bapa,' she said. 'It is not time.' Some water and a trip to the bathroom delayed the coming day.

He had faded in the morning. Alarmed, Mella called Nurse Mary. Things were being set in place, positioning for a march to a faraway place. Mary came in and confirmed a fading blood pressure, a racing heart, poor breath sounds and diminished air entry at the base of the right lung.

Pneumonia, she thought. Mella called me. Pneumonia, I agreed. A tug of memory reminded me that pneumonia was a painless way to leave. Yasmin, my sister-in-law in Freeport, decided to drive down with me to Mella's home in the Pennsylvania hills. His three daughters-in-law gathered around him.

His usually voracious appetite was gone. Not even a sip of juice. Water, water through a straw. Settled on his comfortable left side, a favored and favorable position. How many many pregnant women I have told "left side is best.' Curled on his left side. A circle almost around the world that started as an adventurous young man from a village in India via Africa to the New World was ending.

We announced our presence. He greeted us and we kissed him. There was strength in that old back as he hoisted himself up and asked for water. A wrinkle of hope. "Ya Ali, ya Ali," he said with each breath.

Memories of deaths in hospitals. Aggressive wrenching affairs. With no mercy, no letting go. Traumatic bloody things with tubes and needles and medical violence. He was dehydrated and had pneumonia. Antibiotics and fluids would prolong this day. But we wanted, he deserved, a gentle passing. No, no more. It had been a long, long time. His sons and daughters agreed. They were all miles away in Vancouver gathered for an important birthday. Amir was at a conference in Chicago. Only Bahadur was with us, but the looming death tormented him and he could hardly enter the room. They all agreed to keep their father at home. They agreed, not definitely and boldly, but whisperingly. His understanding family doctor also supported the decision.

The decision was a hurdle. The last hurdle. And then calm. We formed a triangle around him. Mella kneeling on his left, Yasmin seated on his right and I lying across his icy feet. It was a reflection of this man's life that he had emissaries from Europe, India and Africa assembled around him at his death. It was a testimony to him that those emissaries were from wildly different religious faiths—Catholic, Ismaili and Zoroastrian-turned-atheist.

Softly, softly we stroked and held. We kissed and talked. We asked him where he was going. Mella spoke of an earthy paradise filled with his dearest friend—his wife of many decades who had left three years before. A paradise with *kuku paka* and warm *chapattis* awaiting, delicaces from African coast and Indian lands that his wife had delighted him with.

We made room for his only son in presence, one of nine. He was timid, apprehensive of death. He kneeled by his father, held his hand and thought life into him. Dear son, it is too late for what you are thinking.

He left and we reformed our pyramid. Our fragile pyramid. Yasmin, fragrant jasmine flower, on one side, I and the scent of narcissus strewn at his feet. But all he wanted on the third side was his Irish rose. Mella, Mella.

We decided to change him. Clean dry clothes had to feel good. This delicate body was heavier than we anticipated. But his skin was soft and even. A skin well loved and tended. Fine clean nails, clipped just so. We turned and heaved. It was not as easy as we had thought. An extra pair of hands appeared. Carol, Mella's and Bapa's friend, was standing back in the shadows, ready to help when needed. Suddenly it was rapidly done and he was back on his comfy left side.

Icy extremities and overheated torso. How to make him comfortable? Mella said, 'Change the blanket—a lighter one.' Grateful for any purpose, we changed the Western-styled comforter for a bright blue and brightest red blanket. What did he look like? An ancient chieftain. A warrior whose battles were done.

Cheyne-Stokes. Cheyne and Stokes described this terminal breathing. Hyper- ventilation alternating with shallow breathing. He was troubled and upset by the deep breaths but was quiet in the intervals. He started singing a hymn in unfinished words and broken threads. Yasmin took on the burden and completed it for him.

Ya Ali agisani, ya Ali adarakani,
Harbala tu dur kar
Mushkil ashan Ali.

He was asking for forgiveness for sins he had never committed.

A change. The deep breathing did not perturb him any more. Yasmin whispered into his ear, 'Bapa, Bapa.' He did not care anymore. She sprinkled cool water on his forehead to welcome him to this other place. A chant and a beat started and ended days later when they finally covered his aquiline face.

Four weeks later we assembled at his last home, Mella's in the Pennsylvania hills. Driving down from New York, we saw carpets of lime green wild euonymous, and the black locust trees were in bloom, mysterious native trees that bloom erratically every several years. Deep dark black trunks with piles of peachy white perfumed flowers. Masses and masses of them. Why did they bloom this year? We grasped at any comfort we could get.

We played and talked and remembered. We ate and drank and remembered. We said goodbye...and remembered.

And now the living. My children.

Rushna spearheaded going into the 'grown-up' schools. The public school system in the town where we lived, Garden City, was economically segregated and Rushna was practically the only non-white person in school. She tried hard and sometimes crazily to conform, often unhappy with her academic standards that excelled and made her yet still more different from the masses. She went on to Tufts in Massachusetts and law school in Washington. At Tufts she met Kevin Heneghan, whose several generations had gone to this school, and they were married soon after she finished law school. Kevin's father is big Jack who married the football coach's beauteous daughter. He owned but then sold several McDonald's franchises on the New England coast. Kevin's early summers were spent turning hamburgers, which he still does perfectly. Faith, his mother, is now a retired schoolteacher who is the most athletic of women—tennis player, swimmer, ski enthusiast, coach. Also bird watcher and reader.

After four years at Tufts, where his career sounded alarmingly like Amir's, Kevin trained as a software engineer and has held a succession of demanding positions. He is king of hobbies and has gone through fish-rearing, rocket-making, and carpentry, including making guitars—beautifully curvaceous things, crafted from perfect woods. And he makes music on these to lift low spirits.

Children followed and Ellis Amir is now a middle teenager. The kindly and beautiful Cody is just entering his teenage years, and the all-rounder Sierra is a decade old and her mother's principal friend.

Cena's time was softened by the path having been traversed by her older sister. She would always be a city girl and went to Barnard College in New York City. After her master's in sociology, she entered the 'Teach for America' program, a sort of Peace Corps for teaching the underprivileged in the U.S. She selected a school in Brooklyn in the then-bombed-out Bedford-Stuyvesant area. She had her rewards but also her frustrations. A reexamination convinced her that medicine might provide better access to what she wanted.

By this time she had met David Pechefsky at the home of a mutual friend. David's father was an artist and his mother an English professor. For some years after college David worked as a guard at New York's Metropolitan Museum in the Islamic miniatures section. Most other 'career' guards yawn and joke their lives away amongst priceless art. David made the miniatures his backyard with intimate knowledge of the moods and intent of these exquisite paintings.

After graduate work he joined the city council dealing with housing and budget issues and has climbed that ladder to where he now wears a suit and tie to work. He is able to use his intimate knowledge of New York—they are real New Yorkers, he and his family. No car, public transport, bicycles and lately a bicycle rickshaw for pleasure. Bright red in color, the only one in Brooklyn. It has become one of the diversions there, to see him take his family, his mother, for rides in Prospect Park.

Cena and David were married at our home in Ossining. There followed the birth of the extraordinary Tehmina, named after my mother. Cena redirected through the Columbia premed program to medical school at the Downstate Medical Center in Brooklyn. We, who were committed to paying for our children's education, made the last payment for her medical school before we made our last trip to Mumbai. She was to graduate the next spring, and Amir and I as doctors could 'hood' her at graduation. We argued about who should do it—but when the time came there was only I.

She entered a three-year pediatric residency program at NYU and during this work-filled time, had a second daughter—Shirin, Farsi for sweet. Shirin the sweet.

And my passionate Sharyn. Top of her class and forever the defender of the undefended. One of a very few public school entrants to her Yale class, followed by a spell in Teach for America. She was appointed to McAllen, a Texas border town, teaching the children of migrant farm workers. She hurt and suffered through the fact that many children joined late in the school year because they were helping their families bring in the farm produce. That the little child's hand, if viewed alone, appeared adult—larger than it should be and calloused. She did not enjoy this time and returned to go to Georgetown Law School. There on the *Law Review* she met Jon Philip (JP) Devine, whose parents astoundingly were from Marshfield, Massachusetts, a few minutes away from where Kevin's lived.

Sharyn entered the civil rights section of the Justice Department but left in 2000 when George W. Bush was elected to office. After some years with the Feminist Majority, she is back in a government agency to investigate and protect family benefits and rights. JP is an environmental lawyer who started in the government Environmental Protection Agency. He, too, left when Sharyn did and now works for the National Resources Defense Council, an environmental group in the same league as the Sierra Club. I seriously feel safer sleeping with these two fighting for our planet and our rights.

They have Kiran, immersed in books from preschool, though a graceful and natural soccer player, and hazel-eyed Amir with a big big heart.

Years ago, discussing the racial tensions in the Americas, someone suggested that Jamaica's success lay in intermarriage between races. I visualize the peoples in this world slowly becoming light chocolate milk brown, a golden color that all my grandchildren are. Certainly marriages, births and deaths make an adopted country one's own. And what of Africa. Africa. It is not fashionable any more to lay things at the door of the colonials of old. But it is a fantasy of mine to imagine what might have been without the importation of Western religions and political methods. I cannot help but think that local and spontaneous growth might have been brilliant. Brilliant without the importation of British manners and systems, the relentless Belgian thirst for rubber and ivory with a civilized veneer. The world is now flat, we are told. We are all flowing into each other. But Africa has its own genocides, its own military despots, its own leaders who will not give up power or wealth. Its own AIDS. And its own maternal mortality.

Motherhood is a dangerous disease in Africa. The maternal death rates are the highest in the world and frustratingly no different from the '60's when I was there. And this is without AIDS deaths.

Do I have the energy to even think in that direction?

Among the causes of maternal deaths, lack of timely, safe cesarean section stands out. Cesarean section rates are 30% in the U.S. but low, possibly 8-10% in African countries. Is there an ideal rate? No answer. But if cesarean sections in appropriate cases were available, it is difficult not to conclude that maternal lives would be saved. And it would probably reduce the occurrence of the dreaded obstetric fistula, the result of long, neglected labor, which causes so much suffering and makes the woman a social outcast because of her constant uriniferous odor.

But who is to perform these cesarean sections? There are nowhere near the numbers of doctors or obstetricians needed, many lost to medically acquired AIDS and to the brain drain. Primary cesarean sections are simple procedures, and there have been programs to train paramedical personnel to perform surgery. These programs have been long—three years for a program in Mozambique to train medical assistants to perform all forms of emergency surgery—not just cesarean sections.

But three years is too long and, shortsighted as it may seem, I have this fantasy of a plan to train non-physicians only in primary cesarean section, a simple procedure. And train them fast.

Cesarean section has been simplified to bare bones. Let me teach it to you. Incise skin, fat, fascia through a low transverse incision—the popular 'Bikini cut.' Enter the peritoneal cavity. Expose the lower part of the uterus and incise the shiny peritoneum covering it. Push it away and enter the uterus through a wide transverse incision. Deliver the baby levering the head first with your hand. All this takes less than five minutes. After the placenta is delivered, stitch the uterus closed in one layer and the abdomen with a single fascial layer. The days of fastidious complicated multiple layered closure have long gone. This simple closure heals as well and is as strong as the longer techniques. Stitch the skin closed. Do a good tailor's job here—remember this is the only thing the patient sees. I cannot help but think that this can be taught to anyone.

Perhaps I will be able to close the circle of my African life and be allowed to do this.

EPILOGUE

After forty-two years, I lost my friend, partner, lover, companion and playmate. I trace our life together through the beds we have slept in. This was written three decades after my African life ended.

A lifetime of beds - A love story

The first time, I lay on a narrow sagging bed belonging to an Ob/ Gyn resident. The room was closet-sized and on the maternity floor.

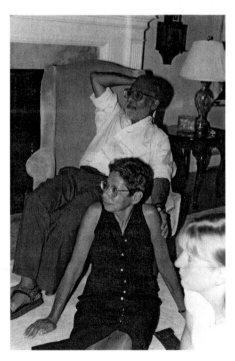

It was 2 a.m. and she, the resident, was away on call. 'Call' here was brutal at 15,000 deliveries a year, 'on-call' lasting a week at a time, night and day. No Bell Commission Rules to temper this. There was no chance of seeing her for the rest of the night.

He sat by the bed and we spoke. Nothing in the biblical sense happened. And yet, looking back, a commitment had started. Did I recognize its sweet shape even then? I remember returning home in the early morning, refreshed, without a second of sleep.

A year later, on yet another creaking old hospital bed on yet another maternity floor, we clung together and said goodbye. He was to leave for Africa and I stayed to complete my residency. On a worthless two rupee note he wrote his address. PO Box 30235. Two and three makes five. Five minus two is three. Add it all together to get thirteen, the size of our family when he finally left us.

A year later he returned and we wed. The twin beds in the hotel where we spent the next month were dragged together and there was an enormous gap between them. *Kapa*, we called it. In the years to come, many twin beds later, we always laughed about who would sleep on the *kapa*. He did. He was better padded and less likely to fall through the crack. On that first night he pronounced me a virgin with a vengeance. My love life started that night – not a moment before we were married—and ended a couple of nights before he died, in Cochin—after a lazy paddle through the backwaters, where we watched the river people make a life out of fish, coconuts and mussels. The last time was on an ornate carved brocaded canopied bed fit for any Amir.

After we were married, we made the crossing to Africa in a P&O ship, the SS Karanja—first class passengers, our wedding present from my father. The cozy wooden bunk beds were a haven because the rest of the passengers in that class were Britishers who did not acknowledge our presence. Passengers from the second and steerage classes, Indians as we were, glowered at us. Too much time in our cabin resulted in a miserable urinary tract infection. Pleasures do not come without their pain.

We were greeted at Mombasa Port by Amir's cousin Mohomedali, who drove us to his home in the Indian quarter. The cousin and his wife allowed us to sleep on their bed in the only bedroom, while they and their children camped out on the floor of the dining/living room. Soon after we had said goodnight a long line of bedbugs streamed out of the crannies of the bed. Bedbugs have a peculiar smell that I recognized before I saw them. This familiarity came from having worked in the 'charity' wards at teaching hospitals. Our first bed together in Africa ridden with bedbugs.

Upper and lower bunk beds on the railroad journey to Nairobi and then Kampala. A memory of fluffy beddings laid out by unseen hands while we were in the dining car while silent and deep Africa sped by the windows of our compartment.

We were to live in his mother's home in Kampala, Uganda. Twin beds pulled together again. That constant *kapa*. We occupied the only real bedroom with eight sibs herded together in the other bedroom. Eight sibs, mother, father and numerous household servants. Not the cozy private life I had imagined.

I entered an Internal Medicine residency and on nights when I was on Emergency Room duty, I was required to stay in the hospital. The call room was on the second floor of the Emergency Room. It was a long hall-like area that ran above the entire length of the ER. Someone told me it had once been a morgue. The only piece of furniture was a bed at the far end of the room, unlike any I had ever seen. It was at least eight feet long and no more than two feet wide. Its most distinctive feature was its height—chest high for both of us. We were at a stage where we could not possibly be separated even for a single night—in any case, there was no way I could get on and off the bed without help. He would push and shove me up and then hoist himself in. We had to cling together on the narrow bed to prevent ourselves from falling out—a deadly possibility at that height. I sometimes think that the forced closeness of those nights cemented something in our lives.

We finally rented a little blue apartment of our own. A real tea-for-two apartment, and we had a bed made for us. Simple as simple could be. Four very short legs and a spring mattress—a reaction to our suicidal Everest bed in the Emergency Room. This bed went with us to our first house, a posting in Jinja as the obstetrician/gynecologist in charge and then back to Kampala where I ran my private practice till we left Africa. This bed stayed with us through three children, who often shared it with us.

We started with residencies in New York. A year after we arrived Idi Amin told the Asians in Uganda to move, and one day they locked their houses and flew to New York. Our tiny residents' apartment now housed thirteen people. A sister, her husband and two children in one bedroom. Mother and father and two sibs in the other bedroom. At a decent time at night, I would encourage our extended family to retire and shut the doors on them. Then Amir, I and our three children laid out mattresses on the floor of the living/dining room and slept calmly and well. I remember those days as needy and busy but glowing.

We started the climb into suburbia and the middle class. Our bed now boasted a plain headboard. Slats and a firm sponge mattress gave us luxury as never before–except that the queen-sized mattress was larger than we were used to. We gravitated to my side and occupied no more than our two-foot Emergency Room bed. The suffering slats on my side would bend and come off their mooring. 'Why my side?' everyone would ask. 'It's her enormous weight,' he would explain. Even now the slats on my side give way. His dark silent weight is still with me.

In a faraway grave at the foothills of the Himalayas, my mother lies with irises thrusting out of her breast.

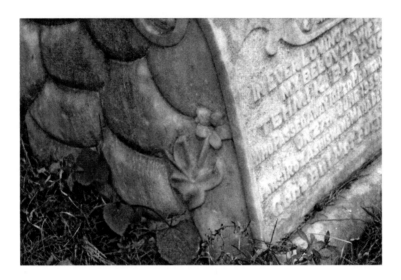

Are you calm in a bed of nasturtiums, spirea, phlox, artemesia, mint and chamomile? Under a quiet apple tree? I am waiting on the granite bench.

CPSIA information can be obtained at www.ICGtesting.com
Printed in the USA
BVOW041911230512

290952BV00001B/12/P